The Tao of your psychotherapy practice

is a way to tune up your practice
with an elegant approach
so your clients
and you
attain freedom simultaneously

When you use the power of harmony with the Tao, you can leverage small steps into large results.

- You will not have to fight insurance companies
- You will concern yourself with neither the size of your practice nor any other mercenary concerns
- You will be able to ride both the forces aiding and the forces hindering your career toward offering your best work for others' benefit
- You will also learn that they will take care of you in return

The world is always moving and renewing, offering us forces to harness—if you know how.

> *"Be assured that there is no question that it can be done. Using these exact methods, I have continued to regenerate a fully independent practice for decades, regardless of economic cycles. Without participation in any managed care panels and without discounted fees, I have enjoyed a full practice of thirty-four sessions each week since I opened my practice in 1986."*
>
> — Rick Blum

Published by The Paradoxical Press, Teaneck, NJ

Please visit Dr. Rick Blum at www.dr-rick.com

Please visit The Paradoxical Press at www.theparadoxicalpress.com

Library of Congress Cataloging-in-Publication Data

Blum, Rick, 1949-

The tao of your psychotherapy practice : how to best serve your clients while maximizing your professional freedom / Rick Blum.

p. cm.

Includes bibliographical references.

ISBN 978-0-9786663-0-9

1. Psychotherapy--Vocational guidance. 2. Psychotherapist and patient. I. Title.

RC465.5.B58 2011

616.89'14--dc22

2010052032

The Tao of Your Psychotherapy Practice

How to Best Serve Your
Clients While Maximizing
Your Professional Freedom

Dr. Rick Blum

the paradoxical press

Praise for Dr. Rick Blum

"Articulate and passionately insightful about a wide range of subjects from psychology to science to comparative mysticism, Dr. Blum has the gift of making the complex lucid—without ever drifting into simplistic generalization. Here is genuine warmth and keen intelligence combined—a rare occurrence in our world of narrow specialization."

Vera Schwarcz, Ph.D., Freeman Professor of East Asian Studies, Wesleyan University, CT.

"As I became exposed to Dr. Blum's work, I was delighted to find such an innovative technology to make change possible for clients. I asked him to present his approach to intervention for my graduate students at the University of Connecticut, and they also responded exuberantly to his vision, humor, and enthusiasm."

Jack Chinsky, Ph.D., Professor of Psychology, University of Connecticut

"You have done for therapists what the innovative martial arts teachers did for combat—observed what the great masters do, then break this down into parts so that it can be taught as a series of techniques."

Steve Simmer, M.S.W., Ph.D., Psychotherapist, creator of the "Men and Anger" seminars, Northampton, MA

To Shoshana

For all the faith you have in me

Contents

Continued...

Contents

Acknowledgments

My first thanks are to the thousands of people that I have met because they entered my office as my clients: You have shaped and supported my work, explicitly and consistently. You continue to make my days beautiful, meaningful, and moving.

Tom Sargent: My original psychotherapy mentor and long-term friend. When you answered my phone query saying that you trained "professional peer counselors," I knew I was in for something new and good. I wish you could see this, but trust that you trusted me that I would write it.

Dency Sargent, Cathy Sargent, and Bernadette Kelley: Along with Tom, you took me in when I was floundering, gave me a job, became my second family, and provided the incubator for everything that came later.

Huston Smith: My first dream come true was becoming your graduate assistant in the religion department at Syracuse University. What I could not know is that you would set me traveling in search of the solution to a riddle. Solving it has made a map for me.

Skip Rackmill: In your friendly, accessible style, you skillfully showed me Aikido in motion.

Jeff Zaleski, Parabola editor-in-chief and publisher: I had written, submitted, been printed, but you were the first who made me a writer—you paid me.

Henry Alker and Susan Hale, advisors at Saybrook University: You guided me in finding the elusive psychological terms to describe what I was doing as a psychotherapist. Without you, there would be no words.

Continued...

Arthur Kurzweil: My friend, *chevrusa,* guide, editor, and buddy, I could never begin to describe the meaning of your company along my path. Your friendship has filled my whole world and continually refreshed my days.

Aliza Stein, my publisher: You joined your insight and enthusiasm for my work with your wisdom on how to best present it. You made it happen.

Deborah Wenger, my copy editor: Arthur always told me that you were the unsung hero of publishing. Thank you for proving him correct.

Irene Abramovich, skilled and caring psychiatrist: Thank you for teaching me about the Tao of medication.

Rabbi Mendel Samuels: Through your intelligence, wit, and insight you effectively challenged my assumptions, and thereby brought together my past with my present, never to be severed.

Larry Blum, my brother: Once upon a time, we were most of each other's worlds. You taught me that having a purpose can save a life, maybe two.

Bernard Blum, my father: You were my first mentor in life and my only hero. You taught me to have no patience for pretense, especially in myself, never to put myself above another person, and to make my work into a bona fide trade. I am grateful that you lived long enough for me to know you were proud of me.

Terry Kole, my mother, and her true love Marty Kole, my stepfather: You were respectively my very birth and the only boss I ever had that I really liked, and you have both been my biggest fans. You also both taught me what a true marriage looks like, by having the best one I have ever seen.

Continued...

Arielle, Alana, Daniel, and Adam Blum: My love for each of you is infinity divided by four. You each made every word possible by forcing me to grow up in 1989.

Rose Blum, mother of my quadruplet children: You didn't let anything deter you from achieving their birth.

Micha, Naomi, Hanna, Evan, and Seth: You weren't looking for me, but opened the door anyway, teaching me about new beginnings up close and personal.

Shoshana: My best friend and my mate, my true and only lady, my best editor and collaborator; you complete my soul and fill my heart.

I gratefully acknowledge You, the One, the only Source of our blessings, who makes everything manifest, who has enlivened us, sustained us, and carried us to this moment.

Tao (*daow*), n., (*ancient Chinese*) 1. the philosophical path consisting of harmonizing direction and force. The word *Tao* means *way*, as in the "Way of Harmony" or as in "Way to go!" It is the way that "No way!" becomes "Way!" 2. the *Tao Te Ching*, (classic text of Tao philosophy): water flows without effort, but makes hard stones smooth and cuts immense canyons (paraphrase). *3. the Tao of your psychotherapy practice is a better way to live, as a person and as a therapist. By allowing your caring efforts for your clients to reach their maximum effect, you will realize a practice that takes care of you too.*

Aikido (*eye-key-doe*), n., (*Japanese; origin an Asian martial art*) 1. "the way of joining with the energy." Any method of synchronized momentum. 2. The "do" in Aikido is the Japanese version of the Chinese word *Tao*; the "ki" (the same as the Chinese "chi" meaning energy); the "ai," means "joined together" (literally "together-energy-way" or "way of harmonizing energy"). Aikido is the most active application of *Tao*. 3. to harness the force of one's opponents to overcome the assault and to neutralize an attack without harming the attacker. 4. *in psychological Aikido both a client's suffering, as well as the instinctive avoidance of suffering, are turned to an advantage.*

Preface
Change Happens

You chose a dream career, and you are still right about that choice. Psychotherapists get to spend their days aiming to permanently enhance the lives of others. Of course, by doing so, we are taking on a seemingly miraculous expectation of ourselves.

- In most people's lives, real transformative change is so elusive that common wisdom insists that no one really changes.
- Further, useful strategies fall into distinctly different theories, not so easily integrated with each other.
- Finally, care management guidelines are seldom oriented toward your clients' and your goals of meaningful change, but rather are aimed at brief symptom reduction and treatment termination.

As a result, we need our own treatment as a profession. This awaits us in the form of the practical philosophy called the *Tao. Aikido,* the most responsive form of Tao practice, shows its greatest promise when aiding an outgunned and overpowered individual, which would describe our clients and ourselves in our quests for transformation. The results of this Tao/Aikido approach to psychotherapy practice are that the very currents that could wash away the joy and benefits of our work become the tide that we can ride back up above the waves.

How Now, Found Tao

As you will see, the same approach that helps us as therapists will be buoyant for our clients' lives as well. Reciprocally, by allowing your caring efforts for your clients to reach their maximum effect, you will realize a practice that takes care of you too. As a result, you will find that the Tao of your psychotherapy practice is just a better way to live, as a person and as a therapist.

To grasp the Tao of being a psychotherapist, we can begin with the metaphor of a small single-sail boat. If you've ever had a sailing lesson, you have been coached to understand that the curve of a sail makes the wind go faster on your side than on the other side. Your side faces the direction you want to go. This speed difference in the wind on each side of the sail produces pressure in a forward direction. With such a magnificent strategy, you can move toward the wind and, if you are flexible enough to dance back and forth (called *tacking*), you can even progress directly against the wind. Notice that, in doing so, you are achieving even more than just moving against the wind—you are actually using the very wind that is blowing against you.

Lessons of a sailboat

Our sail metaphor illustrates the unequalled power of dynamic harmony that the ancient Chinese called the *Tao.* The word Tao means *way*, as in the "Way of Harmony" or as in "Way to go!" In this sense, it is the way that "No way!" becomes "Way!" The best direction to go is often with the flow

"Tao" means "the way"

of forces; the Tao method includes the wisdom of finding a groove and riding it. At first glance this looks like the passive reaction of a driven leaf, but this is not a submissive process. The classic of the Tao philosophy, called the *Tao Te Ching,* instead presents the metaphor of water, which flows without effort, but makes hard stones smooth and cuts immense canyons.

The power of moving water thus comprises the central image of the Tao approach—but notice that there is a difference between a wave and a surfer. The surfer has the option to ride the wave, but with an additional vote on where he or she ends up, just as the sailor harnesses the wind. This sailing-surfing-Tao is a subtype of the Way of Harmony and also has an exotic-sounding Asian (in this case, Japanese) name. It is called *Aikido.* The "do" in Aikido is the Japanese version of the Chinese word Tao. The "ki" part is the same as the Chinese "chi" and means energy, as in "essential forces." This leaves "ai," which means "joined together." Thus, *Aikido* means "the way of joining with the energy" of a situation. More precisely, it is any method of synchronized momentum.

The Aikido surfer

When we use the power of harmony with the Tao, we can leverage small steps into large results. This works because the world is always moving and renewing, offering us forces to harness—if we know how. The way it all moves is through the dance of twos: There are two types of energy that flow together inside and outside us, the dynamic movement of "yin" and "yang." These comprise the mechanics of how the Tao works.

Yin, yang and you

We have already learned the basics in science class. Energy is the basis of existence, say the physicists. As it forms the world, energy expresses itself in the rhythm of opposites. The momentum of the Big Bang versus the force of gravity, positive and negative particle charges, circuits flowing from negative to positive, the binary basis of computer language—you cannot look anywhere in the physical world without seeing binary systems. It is the same with our experience of life: pleasure and pain, birth and death, joy and sorrow, good and evil. In the Tao this duality is called *yin* and *yang*. As opposites, yin and yang refer to receptivity versus action, yielding versus creation, expansion versus contraction, and cold versus heat. Sometimes they are also contrasted as male versus female, but this is only in a metaphoric sense. Nothing can exist without both yin and yang elements.

How does this duality matter? The hidden power within yin and yang is that they tend to create each other. As a result, you can have a significant effect on the outside world, even if you are rather weak yourself. Think of that sail again. Below is the most common way the Chinese illustrated it.

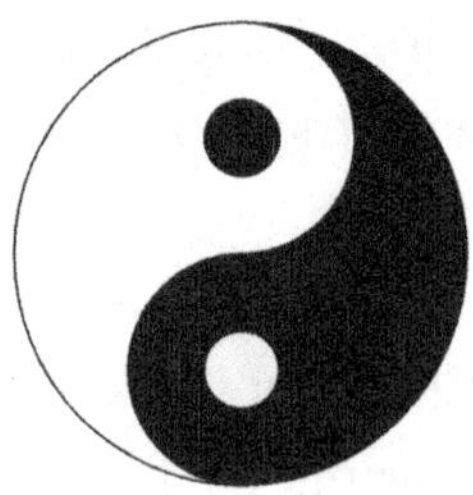

As a symbol, it is familiar and appealing. The *tai chi* (literally "the great energy" and often called the "yin-yang symbol") shows two opposites in the greatest possible contrast, yet enveloping each other to create a perfect whole. Most intriguingly, each opposite, at its very core, *prepares to become the other polarity*. This picture best conveys the perspective on the world called the Tao. Everything is moving and transforming. For this reason, when we are working in harmony with the vibrant reality around us, small actions make a surprisingly big difference. A tiny adjustment in direction results in miles of difference as we travel along. Like the fabled "butterfly effect," in which a tiny winged flutter spurs huge forces when aligned correctly, the "yin" of our sails can take us anywhere when we harness the "yang" of the wind. Then we are in the territory of synchronized momentum called Aikido.

The Tao is intuitive, in that we already sense it within ourselves. This Aikido version of Tao will provide you with the power to use any forces that hinder your practice to your advantage in both helping people and building a superb livelihood. For this reason, its famous application is that of a nonviolent self-defense system. In martial arts, Aikido harnesses the force of an attacker and reverses it onto the assailant. The harsher the attack, the more potent is the reflection. The worse the situation, the more remarkable is the reversal.

How One Trains in the Tao of Psychotherapy

The contents of this book are meant to harness this elegant power in the service of your practice. Our goal will be more than mere understanding—the goal will be to internalize the perspective and make it available to you at will as you help others. In this way, this book is more a workshop than a lecture.

Putting it another way, I am going to provide something of the experience of an Aikido student. The new Aikido practitioner first learns to understand the "power of softness" by watching advanced students overcome opponents with little effort. Additionally, they experience it "up close and personal" as they play the part of the attacker. Then, they gradually absorb the details of Aikido practice.

Mirroring this, our presentation is going to have an unusual organizational structure. We will take this main theme of Tao/Aikido and apply it to three areas: therapeutic strategies, practice strategies, and managing managed care. We have already begun to introduce this, by providing a first pass over the perspective. Beginning in the next chapter, we will explore it more fully, and then we will gradually introduce the details. As we do so, *we will step back periodically and look at the framework, before plunging in again.* Again, this is similar to the way in which a student of the martial art of Aikido is trained. If you resonate deeply with this perspective, and as you begin to reap its benefits, you may find yourself wanting to return to the beginning to approach it again generally before once again getting specific.

Another unusual aspect to our approach to this material, which you may notice, is that we will frequently move between our clients' and our own experiences—and not just our experiences as therapists. In our use of pronouns, we will often describe therapeutic strategies as they would benefit all of us. In fact, you might get the impression that I think *we are our clients.* If you get that impression, you are correct. Although that is not the main theme of this text, woven within the presentation are both the conviction and the rationale for believing that we all share the human condition, and the first beneficiaries for our progress as therapists are ourselves.

The marvelous news about the journey to come is that the Tao of your psychotherapy practice is a way to tune up your practice with an elegant approach so your clients and you attain freedom simultaneously. It means that you will not have to fight insurance companies, and you will concern yourself with neither the size of your practice nor any other mercenary concerns. Instead, you will be able to ride both the forces aiding and the forces hindering your career toward offering your best work for others' benefit. You will also learn that they will take care of you in return.

So, please hop aboard, as we begin.

1

Introduction

The First Aikido Therapist in the West

Perhaps we can learn from the story of a young man whom we can call Jack (a pseudonym, as will be the names in all vignettes to follow). Jack seemed to be a bit on edge, but I could not blame him. His father had shut down emotionally after a terrifying episode during his own childhood and could be a strict judge. Besides, he consistently favored Jack's older brother, who was a powerful and aggressive man. Jack's mother adored him, but this hardly augmented his sense of personal power. Sad to say, he was often viewed as a weakling who was under his mother's protection.

The situation came to a head as his father faced death. Jack and his mother conspired to circumvent the father's wishes for the sons' inheritance. The mother saw a precious gift in Jack, and did not agree with her husband's plans for their sons. Jack, feeling unready to face the consequences, ran away from home as soon as his brother learned about the deception.

In the course of his journeys, Jack grew up. He learned from hard work, from being deceived himself, and from his deep love for a young woman. He married, started a family, and he grew in strength and wealth away from his brother's grasp. In fact, he learned that he combined some of his father's strength of character with his mother's warmth. He also had a remarkable spirituality that exceeded that of either of his parents. Finally, it was time to go home.

On the night before he would face his brother again, he sent everyone away. He spent the night alone—or at least expected to. It was late when he saw the large man approaching him, the man who came to attack him. As the hulking figure came closer, it became clear to him that it was not his brother, but a messenger of sorts. This man had even greater brute power, as Jack soon learned. The man jumped on him, twisting his joints into unnatural positions, squeezing the breath from him.

A night like no other

Despite the violence of the attack, Jack refused to crumble in defeat, though defeat deeply and sorely called to him. Next, the stranger kneed him in the groin so viciously that Jack's hip was dislocated. Throughout this agonizing trial, Jack knew somehow that this was his chance to find out who he was. Surprisingly, he held his own, but certainly not by greater strength. He just decided not to let go. No matter the punishment, Jack held on tightly and tenaciously, squeezing back with all his might. He literally embraced the force attacking him.

Amazingly, the contest went on until daybreak, and its nature began to shift as the sun rose. The stranger began struggling, not for victory, but for release. Finally, he spoke: "All right, then. Enough! Let me go. It's almost dawn!"

An amazing turn of events

Jack would hear none of that, for he had come to perceive that this was no ordinary struggle. First of all, why was he not dead? Also, why did this contest have such a sense of transport to it? Was it the terrific pain and exhaustion, was he dreaming, or both? This moment struck him as the most real of his life, but so different from any other reality in his life. He could not be sure which part of his life was more authentic anymore, either this part or everything else. He was certain only of one thing—this was a sacred point in time, and his tormentor was a messenger to his soul.

It had hit him in a flash of recognition, a glimpse more startling than any of the punishment that the stranger had delivered. The truth of this attack was the climax of all his time in exile. It showed him the core of his life, revealing both a meaning and a mission. This was a truth that could blind a person, could shatter a person's spirit, if it could not be tackled. This stark awareness shouted about the other side of life, about everything we fear, which is as essential to existence as are the parts we prefer. Like a lightning flash to the spirit, the jolt joined above and below. Jack grasped this knowledge both as the most holy and the most ordinary, both as the most hidden and explicit. Now he was unsure if his tenacious holding-on had been a struggle or an embrace.

From this awareness, he spoke his next words: "No! I will not let go of you. This pain will not be for nothing, and I will not have endured only to live. I will not let you go from me without a blessing."

He learns and begins to teach us

"Ya'akov!" the messenger addressed him as Jacob, calling him by his given name. "Yes, you will have this blessing. You are no longer the man you were, and you will not even have the same name as before. Now and forever, you will be called 'Yisra'el,' because you have struggled with the power of men and with God, and you have prevailed."

Yisra'el, "one who wrestles with God"—that is what the name meant. In this way, we read that Jacob was transformed that day, with a new name, a new destiny, and a new reality.

Whatever happened on that desert evening, it became recounted from generation to generation. Translated from the Hebrew Bible, the story became part of the Old Testament, and it still reaches out to us today.

Here we have our own "therapeutic metaphor." Jacob's insistence on a blessing from his travail holds a message for us, both as people and as psychotherapists. The insight has even become a cliché, in the form of the injunction to make lemonade when life hands us lemons. When we consider the alternatives, it becomes obvious that when we must suffer, it would be better to avoid suffering for nothing. Further, if we can wrest blessings from misfortune, we become unstoppable. As life offers us both pleasant and unpleasant realities, once we learn to obtain advantage from the painful events, then nothing can stop our progress. The difference between the trivial recognition of this and the transforming actuality of it is the location of the true challenge.

Aikido in the guise of a cliché

Applying this to professional practice, there are several daily forces working against our goals of best serving our clients while maximizing our own professional freedom:

- Managed care has captured the insurance market, as predicted, so that "private practice" today seems an oxymoron.
- The science and art of psychotherapy is not a "normalized" field—that is, one with a central consensual model. As a result, we can never be honestly sure that we are truly competent.
- Our clients' experience barriers that prevent change, which are stronger than the urges to achieve it.

Our objective together will be nothing less than that of actually harnessing each of these hindrances to the advantage of our clients and our practices. As we will find, the barriers that hinder our building independent and satisfying psychotherapy practices can become the very stepping-stones we climb. Let us take a first look.

Managed care companies want to spend as little as possible on your services. It is not personal—that is their mission. First, they want to convince you that you must either join them or go out of practice. Then, when you join them, they will slash your fees well below what used to be normal in your town. Finally, they will hire you at will—*their* will. If you still cost too much—that is, see clients longer than they like (despite our clients' experience and the suggestive evidence that long-term work is more helpful)—they can fire you. The bottom line: You work for them.

The vise of managed care

This press of managed/confined care aims to imprison practice for short-term company profits. This is unlikely to change; shareholders will expect no less. We, therefore, will expect no more. Instead, we will use this very press as the crucible to develop an adamantine alternative. For example, if you recharge your practice with the power of what we will call a "phenomenal focus," you can both succeed (if you choose) in the private-pay world as well as reinvigorate any of your managed care work with results and satisfaction. This high effectiveness will, in turn, allow you the option to develop an intermittent therapy modality. As we will show, it is possible to be in the financial reach of most people, even if they are out-of-plan, with this model.

The suffocating pressure of managed care will change us one way or another. Either we will huddle together in fear, joining groups whether we wish to do so or not, in order to allow us to join corporate provider-panels, or we will apply the pressure to stimulate an intensely focused and exhilaratingly helpful psychotherapy practice.

This is just the beginning, however. As the managed care vise tightens on our practices, we become underpaid and overworked. On the phone and on my **dr-rick.com** web site, I advise prospective clients about how to pick a therapist off their lists. Half the time, they end up calling me again. When they do, I often hear that they have had trouble even getting the paneled therapists to call them back.

Some reasons to sidestep the vise

Yet who can blame us? We rush to join as many panels as possible, work as much as we can stand in order to make up for severely cut fees, and sign contracts to take the HMO subscribers without prejudice. We are going to be paid as employees, rather than as business owners, no matter how effective we are—yet we will have business owners' expenses. Further, if we are highly skilled, we are just going to get busier, which we cannot manage to be.

The Tao of Aikido, of synchronized momentum, is swift and sweet in coming to your aid. Before you apply any of the other strategies in this text, you can rise to the top of this buoyant wave. Unlike our fellow therapists walled behind the rigid panels, you will offer your clients the freshness and optimism of those who are responsible for and benefiting from their own destinies.

Additionally, the HMOs can actually help you groom your practice style. How is this possible? As you begin to step outside the treatment world that HMOs have created, your awareness of their ubiquitous presence motivates you to work both harder and with more strategic finesse and still fit in those who want to see you. There is no need to hold back, as the fully paneled therapists will have to do to manage their caseloads.

When the vise becomes a devise

You can develop your top capacity as a psychotherapist (which this book will assist you in doing), saying yes to all who want to see you, without becoming unable to fit people in. Some will see the benefits of investing in you; others will not. These sharper folks will choose you and support your independent practice. You will gratefully give back to them wholeheartedly and skillfully. It is a win–win situation.

As a result, even if all else were equal, even if you did not apply any of the strategies you will learn from this book, you will indeed provide a better value service because of these effects. We are gaining a glimpse of how the managed care organizations themselves will help to build your practice, without your joining them. The HMOs, those who present therapists with the lose–lose choice of either losing their practices or losing their own missions, can become your Aikido partner. You see, one's Aikido opponent is simultaneously one's Aikido teacher.

HMO (health maintenance organization), the euphemism that more accurately means "hating my office," can come to mean "how many options" there are for a win–win for your clients and you. MC (managed care), which more accurately means "mangled careers," becomes instead "many contributions"—that is, the contributions you offer through your best efforts and the contributions you receive in return that bequeath your independence.

There are more details, of course. For example, we will sort through the nuts and bolts of setting up an intermittent (time-efficient long-term) therapy modality so it is the most enjoyable and self-maintaining. We will also look at some practice development options.

Managed care is only the most recent challenge for us to transform through Aikido magic. Long before marketing departments invented the myth of the "insurance crisis" (to shroud the financial beating the insurance companies took from the junk bond crisis), psychotherapy labored under its lack of scientific normalization. As a result, some gloriously incompetent therapists can justify everything they do or

Psychotherapy is not normal

do not do based on some untested paradigm. Those of us who care about competence—which includes you—know that we could possibly be making the same mistake unknowingly. After all, it's a catch-22 situation. Few people know that they are insane, and few know that they are incompetent. Knowing this, those of us who care are likely to second-guess ourselves.

To invigorate my practice fully, I must believe that it is worth invigorating. An old adage says, "If you think you can, or if you think you cannot, either way you are right." For my sessions to shine, I must have a basis to believe that I can use therapy time to illuminate freedom and transformation. Yet, as I have pointed out, we are not in a "normalized" science (to use Thomas Kuhn's term from *The Structure of Scientific Revolutions*). Non-normalized fields, such as nutrition, often have dominant models (such as the latest version of the shape-shifting food pyramid), but other models compete heavily. The advantage is a high degree of creativity; the disadvantage is that every approach will receive condemnation by some other audible voices in the field and approbation by still other voices. In contrast, normalized fields, such as medicine, have the reassuring advantage of a consensus about competence, but creativity (for example, the discovery that bacteria could cause stomach ulcers) often suffers.

Because psychotherapy is non-normalized, many of us cannot even clearly articulate our therapy models. Cognitive–behavior theory is dominant in the research, whereas humanistic approaches dominate actual practice. Meanwhile, many other therapists are psychodynamic, behavioral, dialectical–behavioral, neurolinguistic, eclectic, integrative, transpersonal, Jungian, or biological–neurological in orientation. Naturally, all of us will prefer our own model or style of work, or else we would change it; but we can never be certain that we are giving our clients everything that someone of another orientation could provide.

An alternative to this dilemma that will enhance (without replacing) our current models is that of adding a "phenomenal focus."

Introducing a phenomenal focus

The term means a focus on the conscious, everyday experience (phenomena) of our clients, which will naturally engage them as therapeutic allies in achieving rapid change. Another way of putting this is that, in a non-normalized field, you must stay in touch with the confirming data of immediately accessible experience. Of course, this pumps effectiveness into your work, whatever your theory. Thus, through a phenomenal focus, the barrier of theoretical uncertainty becomes an ally. It forces strategic practicality upon us to ascertain our helpfulness. Smile—Aikido is greeting you again.

One example of such readily observed phenomena can be called "state-rigidity" because it refers a state of rigid thinking that occurs during stress. Everyone recognizes this. As I have presented this phenomenon to people for thirty years, to groups as disparate as nuclear engineers and police academy staff, not once has anyone said, "Nope, I don't know what you mean. People don't get rigid and automatic during stress." This temporary state produces a drastic alteration in the nature of problem solving when people move from nonstressful to highly stressful circumstances. We will see how the application of a simple three-step change model can reliably break the rigidity.

A second common phenomenon, which I call "pendulemia," consists of the impasse created by choosing one dichotomy over another. Several straightforward methods are available to rescue clients from dichotomous traps. We will detail them.

Our choice to pay attention to these and other phenomena supplies a practical effectiveness to our sessions without our needing to give up any of our theoretical perspectives. As your clients benefit from the practicality of such a focus, it allows you to develop an accurately good reputation.

Learning not to resist resistance

As for the third challenge, so-called resistance, in some ways it seems remarkable that our clients get any results at all. No one likes to think about pain. After all, pain, by its very nature, is aversive, and our brains have the built-in capacity for denial to protect us against it. Even in the case in which one manages to confront the pain, because of the state-rigidity just mentioned, awareness diminishes just when we need it. At the same time, our clients usually come to us to promote change in their lives, which no one is going to do without the motivation of pain. As a result, people know what to change only when they hurt, and people are usually disposed to avoid knowing that they hurt.

As we are about to see, using Aikido-like strategies, we can best

Before we take a closer look, we should note one important exception. Actually, you can quickly harness the pain that your clients bring to your office to overcome anything but substance addiction. The whole point of such addiction is to further delay the experience of pain, so this retards the process. In this case, we can still eventually help, but usually not alone. That is a big "but," I know, yet nothing in this book is intended as exaggeration or hyperbole. Therefore, the limitations of our efforts are as important to note, as is our potential for excellence. With substance dependencies, you will also often be using support programs for the structure that outpatient therapy just cannot provide. Remarkably, even here, your clients' pain is your greatest ally, as you will ride this Aikido vehicle to "raise bottom" (assist someone in bottoming out in an addictive process without having to spiral all the way down). Further, we will review an Aikido strategy that promotes rapid recovery.

serve our clients by using it all: using pain, using avoidance of pain, and even using resistance to change.

How can we harness emotional pain, when pain either pushes itself out of awareness or engenders a rigid state of narrow awareness? The first step is by harmonizing our clients' and our own efforts, Tao style, by acknowledging that we and our clients are literally in it together. We have already begun to do that. Our awareness of the universality of this dilemma includes ourselves in the picture and moves us gratefully past the "they don't want to get better" judgment. Instead, we can enter our clients' versions of the human condition with the open admission that we share this condition fully with them. We can regard and respect the common dilemma that the aversive experience of pain is necessary as the major source of the motivation to grow. Then we can softly return to the fact that this painful "postman" rings again and again until we answer the door.

As we sit face to face with our clients, we can learn to smile with the confidence that they will answer that door, with us right behind them, and they will open the letter that says, "When the pain of where I am exceeds the pain of where I am going, then I will move." This wise saying has circulated to the point of becoming somewhat of a cliché because, like many clichés, it is true. Seeing the point of the pain, we can apply specific strategies that accelerate the process of applying it. Such synchronized momentum, simultaneously between us and our clients and between our clients and their anguish, is the "way" to which the term Tao refers, and it typifies the most effective way in which things get accomplished.

Such is the type of finesse that will reveal the Tao of your psychotherapy practice, as we move next into the details.

2

How Tao–Aikido Strategies Transform our Clients' Troubles into Allies

Aikido Review

As we have noticed, the term Aikido has its origin in an Asian martial art. Although it may sound like an oxymoron, Aikido is a nonviolent martial art, one in which there are no attacks—at least no specifically Aikido attacks. There could not be, as one needs to harness the force of one's opponents to overcome the assault. The goal in this ethical self-defense system is to neutralize an attack without harming the attacker. The technique is beautiful and graceful, as are all the nonmartial examples of Aikido that we will encounter.

Tao, as we have seen, is the way water yields—but makes canyons. The Chinese term for this inherent power is *wu-wei,* which is translated as "non-doing," as in the classic statement from the *Tao Te Ching,* "Without doing anything, all is done." Paradoxical though this seems, we experience this whenever we see someone doing something so naturally as to "make it look easy." It is the difference between acting and trying.

Sometimes I demonstrate this for clients, as it was shown to me, by asking them to try to pick up a pen. After they pick it up, I point out that they actually picked it up, but could they please *try* to pick it up? Then, I will show how trying looks: a series of false starts and pokes at the

Aikido without really trying

So, how did a Japanese word come to extend to a Chinese concept? Actually, it goes back to India. A classical form of Buddhism that emphasized meditation (dyana, the eighth step along the "eightfold path") entered into China through the 28th Patriarch Bodhidarma. This "Dyana" Buddhism became pronounced "Ch'an" in China. As the name changed, so did this school of Buddhism, which showed a thorough influence of Chinese Taoism. In Japan, this same school became pronounced as "Zen." Japanese culture developed what it received further, as it tends to do, so that we frequently hear of Zen in its influence on culture, philosophy, art, and combat systems.

In Western social science the notion of harnessing and redirecting energy first appears in Freud's concept of sublimation, in which an unacceptable urge is usefully channeled. The psychoanalytic defenses are one of two major Freudian contributions still in widespread use (the other being repetition–compulsion). Aikido provides a positive spin to this notion of sublimation.

Clearly, the Tao symbolism is a rapid and accessible way to introduce the wisdom of harnessing hindering forces to your advantage. Tao and Aikido take form in concrete and naturalistic metaphors. For those comfortable with theological expressions, think in terms of the teaching that all events are planned by God, and therefore ultimately good. In Judaism, there is only God's plan, nothing else, so that every event is part of the ultimate shepherding. Instead of Tao, the Talmudic language is gam zu l'tova. We have already noticed this in the biblical story of Jacob. This also extends to applying one's nature in a useful direction, predating Freud's notion of sublimation. In the Talmud (Shabbos 156a), for example, we learn that a person with an aggressive nature could become a violent thief, or he could become a butcher, a surgeon, or a judge.

In Christianity, we also find this reflected, for example, in C. S. Lewis's concept of God's chisel sculpting our development. As a result, one learns to look for the providential nature of every turn of events. What would be the appropriate response? Aikido would.

pen, while it still lies on the table. Tao-based behavior looks effortless because it skillfully flows with the forces beyond our control, locates the precise opportunities for action, and uses the power of the first to fuel the second. This principle frequently saves lives in the form of the Serenity Prayer of Alcoholics Anonymous (AA): "God grant me the serenity to accept the things I cannot change, the courage to change the things I can, and the wisdom to know the difference." Similarly, as therapists, we learn how effective listening opens up communication.

Aikido arose as an application of the most *wu-wei*-like strategies from martial arts, such as kung fu and jujitsu. As its prowess grew, it inevitably demonstrated advantages in verbal conflict and then in verbal communication in general. The dynamic of Aikido has two essential parts: Align yourself with the direction in which things are already going, and then apply a small amount of effort to change the direction. This is the reason that automobile tires like it better if you let your car wheels roll in the direction in which you do not want to go, before you turn the wheel toward the direction you want. As you are alive to read this, we can assume you also know that you must turn into a skid, exactly toward the danger, to save yourself from it.

Here is a thought exercise that both illustrates the wisdom of an Aikido approach and is a useful example when one explains the model to therapy clients.

Emergency Aikido

Imagine that a child is on a new bicycle but has not practiced with the new brakes, which are hand brakes, not backpedal brakes. The child starts to accelerate down a steep driveway and panics. You see this and feel the same. One choice you have is to run in front of the bike and block it. If you do, the child gets hurt and you get hurt. However, this beats having the child hit the road. So what do you do? You run as fast as you can alongside the bicycle, exactly in the direction that you do *not* want the child to go, so you can take the handlebars and turn them, slightly. The slight movement prevents the child from crashing down and manages to curve the motion onto, say, the lawn.

Clearly, such Aikido strategies have a self-evident quality. They are logical deductions from direct observation of the natural world, as well as from basic physics such as vector analysis.

Psychological Aikido is no different. Seen through the lens of Aikido, both a client's suffering, as well as the instinctive avoidance of suffering, will be turned to an advantage in the strategies to follow.

Whatever works well works this way

Essentially, whatever works best works this way. Specifically, we will see that Aikido helps explain the insight that habits change when we learn how they work and what they want. It is also the way that the best self-esteem strategies work, by achieving what Howard Gardner (in his book *Extraordinary Minds*) calls the "leverage" of existing strengths. Further, by harmonizing energy, even difficult people in the client's life can often be managed effectively—for instance, by aligning one person's goals with the wishes of another, contentious person.

To extend a pop metaphor: the Force is always with you, when you are with the Force. To use still different terms, once you are in sync with the energy of a situation, you begin to get a vote in the direction the situation goes.

The view from a knife

Because our Aikido metaphor springs from a martial art, a thorough look should include this aspect. Here is a glimpse of how Aikido looks when it deals with a physical attack, expressed in the form of a pointedly graphic word-picture. I wrote this after experiencing my first Aikido class. The first exercise presented the harrowing context of having a knife to one's throat. The teacher (Skip Rackmill of Simsbury, CT) immediately helped me to see that, in such a physical confrontation, a type of softness could show extraordinary power, just as I had already learned in my therapy practice. Here is how the image of such an attack and the Aikido response presented itself to me:

Peace is missing, as his lips retract;
His teeth biting into the space between you,
And his knife thrusts forward,
Toward the soft place of your voice,
Beneath your face.
Pivoting, now aligned fully, you are not there,
Not where the knife now pierces air.
Riding his wind, you are with his hatred and his hand,
Now turned in his direction;
Your arm along his,
Your power sitting on his;
A little more even than he offered,
And now he stumbles forward beside you.
Together, in motion,
So that, just another turn, a shift in angle,
And, the way wrists go,
Says he's down.
And his knife is now yours;
So you leave with it.

This is meant to convey some of the flavor of this approach, using the forceful example of a potentially lethal attack. Much less threatening, but also important, are the moments of potential transformation shared with clients inside the privileged space provided by their trust in you. They

Aikido steers therapy between "hmm" and "aww"

interrupt busy schedules to fit in an appointment with you, part with financial assets in exchange for your time, and then present you with the puzzle of some place in their lives in which they are stuck. Your job is to usefully get on board.

For instance, Aikido allows you to escape the extremes of "hmm" and "aww." Therapists tend to swing between being disdainful judges and granting enabling absolution. The first stance opposes the client, whereas the second rides along without steering. To begin with "hmm," if we succumb to the cynical role of judges, we inwardly shake our heads at the follies of our clients.

"Hmm … [wonder how he came up with that ingenious move!]"
"Hmm … [you did *what*?]"
"Hmm … [I told you so.]"

Conversely, others of us prefer to resonate with clients, agreeing that their troubles are never in any way their own doing.

"Of course you felt that way [*aww*, poor thing!]"
"Your good intentions are being misunderstood [*aww*, but I understand you!]"
"How long can you put up with that? [*aww*, I'll rescue you.]"

In contrast, you are operating with Aikido when:

- ☯ You agree only when you sincerely can.
- ☯ At the same time, you guide your clients to see new options for response-ability that are consistent with their goals.
- ☯ As a result, your overt statements can exactly match your private thoughts.

You already do this, when you are most in sync with your clients, Aikido-like, rather than pushing or pulling them. Going along with their energy state, you feel with rather than for your clients, finding yourself saying:

> "Yes, that sounds like it was very painful."
> "It seems like they did not understand what you meant."
> "That type of response from your spouse is not going to work for either of you."

Thus aligned, you can then supply a new direction, as the above statements lead into:

> "Let's find out what else you could have said."
> "If we explore what your goals are, we can sort out a few options that might work out better for you."
> "What do you suppose your spouse would have thought was going on?"

When you operate this way, you are rolling with the mood and perspective presented to you, but then turning the direction only slightly, while still leveraging the existing motivation. This becomes a reliable source of power in your sessions, consistently tapping the power already existing in each client's struggle.

Of course, not all sessions will be worth including in your memoirs. Still, some ought to be. And if not, I promise that you are trying to stand against the forceful waves of personal history, which are throwing your clients where they do not want to go. Change does not happen that way, or at least does not happen best that way. So, whether in combat or counseling, in driving or development, inside or outside, the same question awaits us: go with it or against it? To achieve the kind of continually renewing results that makes an independent practice grow from within, hop onto the situation as it is. Then, look around, and find out what steers it.

How We Can Harness the Obstacles to Private Practice

As we began to see in the introduction, Aikido is also an excellent metaphor for the most effective response to manage our practices in the context of managed care. Nonetheless, this is not a business book! We are going to emphasize the reason for this point more than once. Of course, it is necessary to make a living, but you will not have to try to do so. As will become increasingly clear, the Tao of your practice is such that, by taking the best care of your clients, they will return the favor. Therefore, when bringing up external barriers such as managed care, it is valuable to realize that our focus is not to fret over this threat. On the contrary, we just do not want to miss the opportunity to leverage any of the forces at play, especially the opposing forces. They tend to be especially powerful allies when channeled correctly.

How to succeed in practice without really trying…

We will revisit this important element of harnessing the pressure on practice in more detail in the last chapter. It is important to pay our respects here as well, though, especially in light of the potential effects your independence—if you choose to declare it—will have on both your effectiveness as a therapist and the type of clients with whom you will be working.

The question of in-plan participation is a quintessential Aikido challenge. As our practices are increasingly challenged by the business needs of insurance companies, either we will fight a superior force with an inferior force, or we will leverage the energies of the market changes for our advantage. The attempt to fight force with force would require holding back the movement of large corporations. That is not a tank you want to stand in front of—at least not alone. However, the essential strategies in this text actually originated as a result of these very same marketplace changes. As a result, this Tao approach to your psychotherapy practice will provide greater benefit the worse the practice environment gets.

The obstacles to your practice can, paradoxically, prove such a hidden boon that the benefits actually begin unconsciously, as they did for me, as an accidental side effect of HMOs and preferred provider organizations (PPOs). The positive changes in my practice had their genesis in my working in an Aikido manner with the strange mutations going on in the psychotherapy environment around me. Only later did I realize that my adaptations had fortuitously inoculated me from the damage.

This applies to you also. Capitulation to your fears over HMO dominance will create an adverse effect on your ability to help the rest of us, especially as we are asking you for help with our own fears. Breaking free of that dominance, whether suddenly or gradually, has a much different effect. Those who engage this challenge effectively, in an Aikido fashion, will radiate enthusiasm and confidence. In this way, the Tao of our psychotherapy practices renders us the best therapists we can be, precisely because we lack any other choice that includes independent survival.

No choice but excellence

For this same reason, people in AA often work harder than do your clients in other twelve-step programs. Because they have come to believe that they must either recover or die, they know that they have no choice but to "work the program." Similarly, we have no choice. We will each become our best, not only because we want to, but also because the changes around us have caused us to see that we either conduct our own practices exquisitely or suffer the death of our dreams as therapists. Such a dramatic contrast can really wake you up.

Once we fully alert ourselves to the task, the HMO and PPO panels will even keep our caseloads manageable for us. We can just show up at our offices, engage fully in sessions, offer our best work, without the fear of becoming busier than we can stand. Let me explain how this works.

Surprisingly, it is simpler than it looks

Everyone who calls me, whether from the yellow pages—where about 10 percent of us remain—or from personal referrals, receives my best efforts. I either help to answer their questions and schedule a meeting, or do my best to guide them in picking someone from their insurance company's provider list. I have two pages devoted to the subject on my web site. The first recommends that people choose someone out-of-plan, and the second guides people in how to choose someone else.

Here is where one can see the full elegance of Aikido harmony with the external challenges around us. *I get a call back only from those sharp enough to realize that a therapist who is so helpful to a complete stranger is the right one to see.* As a result, most of my clients are my favorite people, and they would be wherever I would have met them. They are bright, committed to growth, and eager to assume responsibility for their lives.

- ☯ They tend to be highly intelligent because they easily understand that there are more elements involved in assessing their investment in psychotherapy than the single factor of their copay amount. They figure out that there may be an important reason that I can stay out-of-plan.
- ☯ They are usually committed to growth and eager to assume responsibility because those who are looking for a "resonating" therapist (a yes-man or yes-woman) will run for the hills

when they encounter a practice that is strategically rich and oriented toward transformation.

In this way, HMOs/PPOs and my practice approach combine to become the filter that brings the most satisfying clients to meet me. What a way to spend my days! Being helpful is my part; the rest of the selection process is managed by the insurance panels that I do *not* join. This is the option that we are beginning to make available to your practice as well.

In this manner, Aikido becomes a central metaphor for the independent practice of the future. The existence of the practice style in this text owes its leverage to the destructive aspects of managed care. The fervor with which we apply it will benefit equally from that same pressure. In other words, pressure can stimulate effectiveness, if it is at the right level (as the inverted-U studies always show, for example, Broadbent 1971; Duffy 1962; Kemeny 1979; Zajonc 1965). The most potent combination for high performance is that of stress plus confidence. This produces the "flow" state (Csikszentmihalyi 1990), in which performance is at its best. Finally, the therapeutic Aikido-like strategies, which we are about to review, will infuse our sessions with a "phenomenal focus," with unassailable power.

A new metaphor

In this way, the Tao perspective allows us to have vibrantly successful practices without becoming overly business-oriented. In fact, these principles suggest that we will "do well by doing good," as the expression goes. None of the elements of the previous paragraph requires a mercenary focus. Quite the contrary—such an emphasis would only interfere with the high-performance "flow" state. This is terrific news.

Because you are a helper, as I am, we would both rather talk about therapy and transformation than business and money. The win–win situation is that the first of these produces the second. So let us now turn to the Tao of therapeutic technique.

Aikido Puts the 'There' in 'Ther-apeutic'

As we begin to look at the surprising therapeutic power of the Aikido version of the Tao, it is a good time to stress that we are not replacing whatever paradigm you currently like to use in your work. Instead, we are applying the useful effects of the readily evident phenomenon of Aikido, which is the difference between fighting force with force and channeling the energies already present in any situation. Later, we will consider how such strategic excellence coalesces with various models. At that time, we will also see how to overcome the obstacle presented by psychotherapy being a non-normalized field (lacking a consistent consensus on a single model).

Because Aikido originates in a martial art and performs conflict resolution quite effectively in that arena, the most natural application of Aikido to psychotherapy is in verbal conflict. This has prompted several books on the subject, such as *Giving In to Get Your Way* by Terry Dobson and Victor Miller and *The Magic of Conflict* by Thomas Crum. In this section, we will explore applications to the overall psychotherapy, as well as including a section on verbal self-defense.

All the strategies we will discuss have in common a refreshing emphasis on starting exactly where we are. Perhaps this suggestion seems so obvious as to appear facile—yet it stands in strong contrast to how people typically attempt to grow and change. Paradoxically, we want to scramble away from where we are in such a hurry that we often cannot

You can't get there from here

gain our footing. Instead, we dig ourselves into a rut, so we become stuck in the exact place that we hate. When we thus spin our wheels, we do the same with the emotions we already have: We feel anxious about our anxiety, guilty about our guilt, angry about our anger, fearful about our fear.

The last thing that people want to do is to accept their starting points. That is why they want to change; they do not like where they are. Without initial acceptance, though, there is no awareness. Without awareness, we are stuck with guilt and/or blame, often alternating between them. In the context of intense guilt or blame, no change occurs. Thus, I often find myself saying to clients:

> You know, if you wanted to get to that door and you couldn't start from your chair, but you had to start from another chair, you could never leave! You'd have to spend your entire life in that chair. You can begin moving only from where you already are.

At moments like those, no one rejects my point as excessively tautological. Thus, the overall formula for applying Aikido strategies to therapeutic change is Tao all the way. It…

- ☯ Begins with acceptance of where life's journey has put one so far;
- ☯ Continues with applying one's dissatisfaction to provide energy for movement; and
- ☯ Energizes motion by finding resources in the current situation that can propel oneself to the next step.

Tao is the 'Way' of Emotional Healing

It is easy to imagine that such a valuable approach can provide a practical advantage in several areas in which we coach our clients. For example, the Aikido approach offers a key to opening the locks that confine people in what we could call "emotional prisons."

Such prisons can be brutal both in their confinement and in their torment. What is such a jail made of? Often, people involuntarily build it out of the feelings that they learn to avoid. For example, depressed people regularly terminate their own lives, sometimes in horrible ways, rather than experience powerful anger, which they have learned is unacceptable. Similarly, rage-prone people often destroy others' lives, and finally their own, rather than experience fear or sadness. A violent man frequently has a prison guard in his head, forcing him to do whatever he has to do, no matter how beloved is the life he harms, in order to avoid vulnerability.

Babies seem to be born with the ability to feel distress in the hues of "mad–sad–scared," three primary distress colors that change our energy state and communicate to others. Subsequent experience changes that capacity, as young children decide "Never again!" regarding a certain emotional response. To achieve this avoidance, people develop complex forms of suffering, such as guilt, resentment, depression, detachment, and anxiety. Many times, the regained ability to have one of the three basic feelings relieves our clients from the captivity of one of these complex feelings–traps.

For this reason, when people benefit by learning new forms of emotional expression, they are simply taking back the innate feelings with which they were born, those that they later exiled from themselves under pressure. Here, Aikido helps people find the right feeling through a process of elimination.

Finding the right feeling through the wrong one

So, rather than fighting the upsetting feeling, we use it. To begin, I can ask myself which feeling—say, anger, grieving, or fear—best describes my emotional state. The best next question is whether that emotion is working to heal me, or whether it is covering up another feeling. In other words, is it a "good cry" or a relieving vent? Am I "getting it off my chest?" If I am expressing some form of upset, either I will feel relief or I will not. If I keep experiencing the same feeling, but do not feel better, chances are I am not experiencing the particular emotion that would hasten healing instead.

Thus, Aikido-like, we can impress the wrong feeling in service toward finding the right one. Rather than our clients judging themselves for even excessive feelings, we can prepare them to ask themselves, "Is this healing me? Does awareness of this feeling give me a greater range of choices in my actions? Does it finish, leaving me more whole?" When the answer is that it does not, we do not have very far to look, as the missing feeling is usually one of the three primary feelings. This strategy is surprisingly effective, especially considering its simplicity.

One situation in which it may not seem to work is when a person has a cycling emotional state. Even here, however, we can flow with the wrong feeling to find the right one. It's just that the prescription for success will change from mood to mood. The requisite emotion for relief will be different in an agitated state than in a depressed state. Again, this underscores our need to accept the place from which we start.

How Aikido Responds to OCD and Phobias

When it comes to emotional prisons, one cannot outdo either the compulsive or the repulsive (phobic) disorders. Obsessive-compulsive disorder (OCD), in its compulsive side, makes a person a puppet. The strings are in charge. They say to go back and check the same door lock again and again, drive back and forth on that same road in case you really did hit someone with your car, or reread this same sentence again and again. The obsessive spectrum is even more draconian, taking over consciousness. One must think the same unpleasant loop repeatedly, so that there remains no room for enjoyment. As for phobias, they render a part of the world terrible. Sometimes the fear is of small creatures, and other times the fear is as large as other people or the world itself.

Owing to the horrible enslavement by these disorders, one can find several popular approaches to treatment. The most helpful will have an Aikido element. For example, repeated obsessions often mask a taboo emotional reaction. At some point many creative, intelligent people come up with an effective way to avoid forbidden emotions and become *too* good at this avoidance. Obsessive people usually have one of the primary feelings kept off-limits. Anecdotally, I have noticed that about 90 percent of my clients are avoiding anger when they obsess, whereas the rest are usually avoiding feelings of loss. This has spurred me to prompt my clients that "obsess" equals "repress."

Another way I find myself expressing the matter handily extends the meaning of a popular expression. While obsessing, people "make mountains out of molehills." Of course, they know this, even as an aspect of diagnosis. They hate their obsessions and usually consider them "stupid." If they believed the content of their obsessions, they would be delusional, not obsessive. To break the cycle, I suggest to these clients, "People make mountains out of molehills so they don't have to think about the real mountains."

The secrets of molehills finally revealed!

This begins the process of returning a choice for OCD sufferers. Either they can obsess, or they can use the obsession as a cue to face the taboo feeling. In this way, the obsessive symptom becomes Aikido-transformed from an "inner enemy," as people initially perceive it. Instead, they begin to see it as an overused strategy with the original purpose of shielding them from unwanted emotional content. Consequently, the presence of an obsession can become a signal for a choice, rather than the occasion for an argument with oneself. It is an extraordinarily simple Aikido strategy of using the symptom as an aid to recovery from the symptom. With repetition, it breaks the open the prison door.

Here is a case in point. Mary comes into my office shaken, because she has had another violent obsession. She was boiling water on her stove and imagined throwing it onto her husband. Never a violent person, she condemns herself thoroughly for such wicked thinking. This only increases the pressure of the obsession. She cannot stop. In our discussion, which follows, what I say is in *italics*.

She says:

"I can't believe I was thinking that! I'm horrible."

Did you think that you were going to do it?

"No. It wasn't like I was reaching for the pot or anything. But, what kind of person thinks things like that?"

A person with obsessions does. Last time we found that you felt angry and didn't know it. Do you think that could be going on now?

"There was nothing to be angry about. That other time he was acting annoying, so what you said made sense. This time he was just sitting at the table. I was glad he was there, so why should I imagine scalding him?"

So, you were completely happy with him this time.

"Well, who could ever say 'completely'? That's a hell of a tough standard, wouldn't you say? I mean, no one's perfect. You know what I mean."

No one I know. So, are any imperfections of Bob's affecting you these days?

"Not right then."

Then, right when?

"Like, the day before."

Like what?

"Okay. I found out he lost more money in his little, expensive hobby."

You mean the stock trading?

"Right."

How'd that hit you, hearing that?

"It's his money. I guess he wants to do more than manage a store some day."

So, it's his money, and you did not mind that he lost it.

"No. I didn't like it."

How much?

"I was a little peeved."

Peeved? As in a little, tiny bit 'miffed'? I think you were miffed last time. Good thing you weren't angry.

"Okay, okay. Shut up."

There we go. How angry are you really?

"He has no right to spend our little bit of extra money on get-rich-quick schemes. Even when the market is good, you lose when you get greedy. I wish he'd cut it out, but he won't listen. I am angry."

How much are you obsessing, now?

"The hot water is gone, though maybe I should throw it on his broker. Only kidding!"

With reinforcement, Mary slowly learned not to fear her obsessions. She began to actually use them. They became her signal to explore what might be angering her. Next, we worked on forms of assertiveness so she could channel her anger effectively.

Turning to the compulsive side of OCD, compulsions bear an interesting similarity to phobias. In both cases, a person feels coerced to act in order to avoid feelings of dread. The clinical term for the OCD version of such horror is "pathological doubt." One must perform an act that becomes addictive because it temporarily lessens one's dread without the need to ever confront it. *In this way, both compulsions and phobias grow by fueling avoidance of a dreaded experience.* In the case of compulsive avoidance, the pressure is to repeat a particular act, whereas in cases of phobic avoidance the pressure is to retreat. Either way, one ends up controlled by the very fear that one is avoiding. Additionally, in both cases, the person feels very foolish. Just this morning, a client laughed as I remarked, "You think you're wacky!" Fortunately, both compulsions and phobias respond to similar strategies.

Aikido in the treatment of phobias

Next, we have a chance to practice recognizing Aikido when we see it. Let us compare two different versions of phobia treatment, both of which are cognitive approaches, using such an Aikido lens. You can decide:

- Which has the most Aikido feel, and
- Which has the most therapeutic appeal.

In either technique, first you must prepare the person to frame the irrational fear correctly. One option is to identify the distorted premises rampant in the "set of anxiety-engendering avoidant thoughts" (Meichenbaum 1977, p. 153). This is state-of-the-art cognitive–behavioral therapy (CBT) and is familiar to many of us. Another option (Bernstein 1999) applies a kind of critical-incident stress debriefing. As it is less familiar, this approach requires a bit more explanation for us to understand it. Looking back at the earliest incidents that formed the phobia, we render them as normal reactions to abnormal situations. The goal is to see that phobias are not foolish, just outdated patterns. Like the rest of our behavior patterns, associations, not logic, connect them. Unlike the rest of our automatic reactions, these patterns hurt us.

Next, the Meichenbaum approach practices "coping self-statements" aiming to rid oneself of the crippling anxiety. One practices or "rehearses" the new statements, with the intention of "inoculating" oneself to the stressful encounters. In contrast, the Bernstein method guides people in the expectation that, in light of the critical incidents, anxiety is predictable and inevitable. Instead of trying to cope better, people develop a one-to-ten anxiety scale and aim to practice exposure at around a level four or five. With repeated exposure, the fives naturally drop to threes. As they do, the sevens drop to fives, and so on. In practice, it can be done with exposure (overtly) or as part of a desensitization model (covertly, in your office).

So, which of these has more of an Aikido feel? Which one works with the force of the phobia, rather than against it? Wouldn't the second approach best ally you and your clients as partners in achieving freedom from crippling phobias? Similarly, when working with worry in general, the best first step is one of Tao alignment.

An Aikido approach to treating anxiety and worry begins with the observation that fear reduces to two words: "what if?" Asking that question is not a bad place to start considering a problem. There is nothing wrong with—and there is perhaps some wisdom to—

The first step to managing worry is an Aikido step

beginning any course of action with assessing the risk. It is just a painful place to finish one's thinking. If we formalize the worry segment as a legitimate part of problem solving, we can more easily move beyond it. Sometimes I will suggest, "Start with 'what if' and end with 'what's next.'" As a consequence of this Tao-like acceptance of the need to start with worry, the anxiety strategies we employ become much more effective.

The Gentleperson's Art of Verbal Self-Defense

Because Aikido strategies stem from a self-defense art, there is little surprise that they can help defend oneself verbally. Dealing with difficult people is "not often easy; it's not often kind" (to apply John Sebastian's lyrics), but these strategies are both gentle and effective. In a physical confrontation, Aikido moves through three phases:

- One pays attention;
- One aligns oneself with the direction of an attack; and
- Then one extends that attack in a direction that neutralizes its aggression.

Taking the same steps into verbal difficulty, we can manage thorny communication in three stages: *listen, assess,* and *steer.* As we move into these listen/assess/steer strategies, our aim is to inculcate the Aikido perspective further, as well as to supply handy treatment options. In most cases, clients will not want or need your presentation of the entire framework. Rather than learning the format, they will usually prefer to have you supply the options that might fit their goals. With that in mind, we begin with the first step, that of listening.

We may have varying goals when we are speaking with someone, and the way the other person is treating us varies considerably as well. All this can be confusing. Fortunately, the first step can be always the same—*effective listening*. The word "listen" is an anagram of the word "silent," and that is the first element of effective listening, but it does not end there.

The technique most often employed as an effective listening strategy is "reflective listening," which is essentially a paraphrasing activity. It is helpful, when compared with not listening, and it has research documenting its role in helping relationships. Still, people usually find this strategy awkward, if not annoying. Through the filter of Aikido, we can see that reflective listening is a little too passive, somewhat more compliant than engaged.

Positive interpretation, which I often call "wishful hearing"

The difference between "reflective" and "effective"

Of course, sometimes we do not even have the opportunity to practice good listening, because the other person is not interested in talking! What would be an Aikido strategy to inspire somebody to listen? Engaging another person in conversation that he or she is avoiding can be a daunting task. Amazingly, I have never known the following solution to fail.

I call the solution a "once–well" conversation because the person offers to address an important subject only once, but well enough that once is enough. Often the other party has no expressed interest in the discussion, so it takes Aikido excellence to engage any attention at all. The force that we will be harnessing and extending is the very fact of such disinterest from the other person. The once–well presentation takes precisely the same point of view, that there is no point in belaboring the issue. In fact, the

Continued on next page

angle of the presentation is an offer to talk about this so clearly that it will be unnecessary to bother with it again.

Here is a sample script introducing a once–well conversation:

> *There's something that I have been thinking about telling you. I think I would regret it if I never mentioned it. I don't need you to agree with me; and I don't even expect that you will. I just want to say it one time and know that you heard me. Then, you can tell me that I am wrong, if you think so. All I will want to know is that you have heard what I said. Does that make sense?*

So, far I have never heard anyone refuse the conversation if it is presented this way. Typically, the other might say, "What is it already?" Just as typically, when one is interrupted immediately upon beginning, it can prompt the following:

> *As I said, I don't expect you to agree. I just want to know you hear me. So if you are willing to listen, I just have to get through it once and then you can tell me what you think.*

This encouragement of disagreement disarms it. Instead, other people will usually listen through the entire presentation and then only afterward explain how wrong you are. When you affirm that you accept the fact that they don't see it the same way and that you just want to know whether they understood your point of view, they will usually commit to that. In this way, communication without an argument takes the wind out of other people's opposition. In its place, it leaves them to think about what you said after you have left.

This once–well approach is one of my clients' favorite strategies—it supplies the serenity of knowing that one has given important information to another person, leaving the use of that information up to him or her. Once the other person is talking, we now have the opportunity to practice effective listening.

in my office, is an example of an Aikido approach to listening, and it addresses ambiguity in communication. Statements, especially those made during stress, are often unclear. Frequently, a person's comments to us can be taken one of several ways. "I don't want to argue with you" could mean "I will work really hard to resolve this effectively with you," or it could mean, "I wish to heck you would stop talking to me!" We are often afraid that the other person meant the remark in the most negative possible way. Of course, we are sometimes correct about this. Still, we are better off interpreting a comment in the best possible light.

"Wishful hearing"

If we act this way when the other person actually meant no offense in a comment, we avoid what Markman et al. (1994) call "negative interpretation," which they documented as one of the chief ways in which people erode significant relationships. On the other hand, if the other person really intended a combative meaning, we still benefit by "playing dumb." Often, this individual has spoken during an upset mood, will feel embarrassed about the original meaning, and will back away from it. Of course, even when people do not backtrack—and even correct you that they meant their remark exactly in the way you had feared—at least you then know what the argument is about and can proceed from there.

A second Aikido listening strategy is that of eliminating negative interpretations, which is especially useful for less ambiguous-sounding and difficult statements. One cannot always pull off wishful hearing. Sometimes the statement one is hearing just sounds too negative; other times, one is just too angry to manage a positive

Eliminating negative interpretation

interpretation. This shows the need for another way to check out one's understanding. This second option of effective listening maintains an Aikido advantage because it still gives the other person a chance to reverse direction. Another way to phrase this technique (which I prefer when teaching it) is, "When in doubt, check it out." As simple as that sounds, achieving it usually takes some practice. The exercise below can accomplish this.

- In the first step, you can direct clients' attention to their bodies as a signal of the need to check out a statement: "Notice the feeling of discomfort in your middle that tells you that you are taking offense."
- Second, ask them to articulate what they think they heard and what it meant to them: "Ask yourself how you interpreted that which you heard. What did you think the other person meant, which in turn created that discomfort?"
- The third step is the relatively simple matter of asking: "Ask the other person if that is what he or she meant."

In the following illustration, the new thoughts you are modeling are in brackets.

Spouse:	"Here you go again. Just when I was hoping to have a good weekend, you have to start."	
Other spouse:	Step one:	[Ouch, I just got zapped!]
	Step two:	[What did that mean? I think it's that I won't let us have a good weekend.]
	Step three:	"Are you thinking that I just won't let us have fun this weekend?"

Of course, sometimes this is exactly what the first spouse meant. Nonetheless, there is often a change of mind after this strategy. People often do not like how they look in the lucid mirror of such effective listening. This is the elegance of Aikido in action. One party's willingness to listen so carefully (and to an argumentative statement, at that!) offers an inviting alternative to that argument. Of course, the other person may not take one up on this splendid invitation. Fortunately, a third Aikido listening option remains.

Accurate agreement

Accurate agreement takes listening to its highest level. In the previous option, one did not show agreement or disagreement, just the willingness to understand. In contrast, accurate agreement seeks to find any areas of reassurance and accord. It is wise to emphasize the "accurate" element of this approach. To express conformity when one does not agree would create a host of troubles. On the other hand, to withhold the expression of agreement, when it is accurate, is to participate in misunderstanding. To return to the previous couple, assuming the checking-it-out strategy had little effect:

Spouse: "Am I thinking that you won't let us have fun? You bet I am. And, why would I? Is it because you find a way to make trouble whenever I want to have a good time? You can bet on that, too!"

Other, more skilled, spouse:

"I agree that there have been too many times when you were looking forward to a good time, and you ended up disappointed. You've mentioned it before, and I'm sure it is true. I want to let you know that I am alert to this, and I am going to focus my attention on our having good times together, including this weekend."

Admittedly, this was a master's level of accurate agreement, and we, let alone our clients, may not always reach that pinnacle of excellence during stress. With practice, however, we can get surprisingly close, especially when we see the power it has to diffuse verbal contention. Once we have expressed agreement, when it is accurate, we have done our part to provide an Aikido standard of active listening. If a conflict persists, it is time to make a move of our own, but that action depends on one's assessment of the situation, as we will see.

To extend our Aikido metaphor, our best move will depend on our assessment of what we are facing and what we would like the outcome to be. This next step is again something that we can do for our clients, rather than something that they would usually need to learn. During this assessment, we determine, first, what the goals of this communication are and, second, what kind of barrier confronts that goal. This probably sounds complicated, but with examples and with our own practice, it truly becomes straightforward. We are really referring to only two questions: *What's the goal?* and *What's in the way?*

Sizing up the situation well

Turning to the first question, we will be finding out in the examples to come whether the goal is intimacy (closeness), neutralization (stopping a verbal attack), or enrollment (gaining cooperative action). The first is about love, whereas the second two are power struggles. As we will see, manipulation is unacceptable when the goal is intimacy. It may seem justified, as the other person is uncooperative even in the face of our excellent listening, but it does not fit a goal of enhancing love. Thus, you may gain capitulation from a friend, but at the cost of some of that friendship.

The second question we will be asking to size up the situation is

"What's in the way?"—that is, what is the nature of the communication barrier? For example, when the goal is intimacy, is the other person being overreactive (explosive), underreactive (distant), or cautiously responsive (afraid)? If neutralization (stopping an attack) is the goal, is the power potentially equal, or is your client subordinate to another? Finally, if the goal is enrollment (gaining cooperation), is there any mutual interest or not?

Much as in a physical attack, our assessment will provide our options for the next step, which is steering the situation in a positive direction. We will see next how this can play out. Of course, I have applied many different strategies over the years, as have you. However, I typically find that the most useful include this combination of going with force and then redirecting it. The strategies I share here happen to be my favorites.

When one's goal is intimacy, the preferable endpoint would be greater closeness. There is both bad news and good news about this goal. The bad news is that we cannot guarantee that our clients' partners will grow. Essentially, we cannot induce other people to grow in the directions we would recommend for them. Even if they would be happier if they followed our lead, that decision is theirs, not ours. No one can make another person reach his or her potential. Unfortunately and paradoxically, though, *we can succeed in making them worse.* How can it be that we cannot make someone better but can make him or her worse? The latter occurs when we supply high stress to the situation. This distresses the other person, or further distresses the person if he or she was already upset. Because of the effects of stress, we can elicit old distress patterns, especially from people who care about us.

Aikido when the goal is intimacy

The fact that we cannot make people better, but can so easily worsen them, seems unfair. The good news is that we are already making them worse, in most cases. This is good news? Yes, it is, because, as a result, it will actually appear as if we are improving them when we change *our own* behavior.

For example, when other people are overreactive, our clients are usually reinforcing the conflict, unwillingly and unwittingly. It is natural to become upset in the company of an argumentative person. Such upset usually takes the form of either placating or arguing back. Either response is usually more intense than whatever otherwise goes on when the volatile party is not exploding. You know what typically happens: Our clients learn to keep their heads down and tend to withdraw in order to avoid trouble. As a result, they are training their partners that their best shot at an intense response is to argue even more, until our clients either explode themselves or vigorously defend themselves. This comprises the reinforcement, and this is what I meant by making the other person worse.

Explosive intimacy

Much more useful, especially after the effective listening outlined earlier, is a simple three-step Aikido strategy that people can quickly learn. In family systems terms, we are advising our clients how to avoid placating a blamer.

- First, you tell the other person *what you'd rather do*—that is, what would be preferable communication; for example, "This sounds important to you—too important to fight about. I'd like to sit down as friends and see if we can sort it out."
- After the other party has heard this quality offer, if nothing changes, the second step is to say *what you won't do,* which

means refusing to continue this argument. "As I said, I'd be happy to talk this through, but I won't be able to make sense if you are yelling or calling me names. So I'm not going to do that with you."

- Finally, if there is still no change, the third step is *a timed break*. This is decidedly different from just walking out. In fact, the gold standard for this step would be to say something such as, "I am just not able to treat you the way that you deserve if I listen to you yelling at me, so I'm going to take a break and be back in forty-five minutes, so that I can cool down and be with you the way I prefer."

The sweet balance of this approach is to listen effectively, offer caring and interest, and then slowly withhold reinforcement of an argument, ultimately removing oneself if necessary. The argumentative force of the other person fuels the desire to escape, and we are directly channeling that into the timed break. The break must be time-limited, however, so the other person knows when one is returning. If this is done without storming out, it completes an effective approach that offers an alternative to argument, without participating in the fight. The angry partners *get something for nothing and nothing for arguing*. They receive a better offer than an escalating tussle and little incentive to stay stuck. Unless the other party is psychotic or drinking, this is ultimately a can't-miss strategy. It truly blew me away when I first started using it, and it still does.

Similarly, if the other party is underreactive, our first goal is to avoid making the situation worse. When another person is emotionally distant, it tends to stimulate the desperate urge to pursue him or her. We all tend to want what we cannot have. So, again, we tend to "pay off" behavior that we hate,

Dealing with distance

when we try to cajole a response from detached friends and lovers. Then, when these people finally come around, it is just as natural to sulk and punish them for their previous distance. Accordingly, the dance goes on.

People in relationships with such "distancers" spend hours analyzing each gesture and expression, as the other person does not say much. They keep attempting to market the importance of communication to someone who seems to find just looking at them as a form of forced labor. How does this feel from the other person's viewpoint? Have someone grab your hand, put on a slight but steady pressure, and not let go. To add effect, ask them to add a sad expression, and say, plaintively, "Please don't go." It starts to feel like glue, and, voila!, you are on the desperate side of a distance-pursuit dynamic. (This is a great activity in sessions, by the way.)

A better, and very Aikido-like, approach replaces our clients' endless analysis with only one simple question. All one does is to ask oneself, "At this moment, is this other person coming forward or pushing away?" One's job of analysis has just become extraordinarily simple.

When it's better to go fishing

When people are pushing away, the most Tao/Aikido response is not to be there for them to push away. To use a different analogy, this is why there is a "drag" button on deepwater fishing reels. No matter how tough the line, if the fish is powerful and adamant, you break the line when you put force against force. So, returning to human communication, you offer even a bit more space than the other person has asked for.

An example of this is, "Of course you're right that we may not end up together—and, in fact, the direction of things looks kind of negative at the moment, doesn't it?"

Or, "Yes, I can see that you have a lot to do, and so you can't tell me what time you'd be coming over. Maybe it would help if you just took the time to get that stuff done, and we can assume you won't be coming over today."

Conversely, when these people begin to return, whether in anger or affection, one gently receives them, reeling them in steadily and gently. The point of this combination is that of warmly reinforcing the other person's slow approach, while giving nothing for distance. This does not change the other person. If the other person does not care or has another lover, nothing will help. This strategy simply removes oneself as a negative variable and allows the other person to experience caring, if it is there. As singer-songwriter Bonnie Raitt put it, "Love has no pride, when there's no one left to blame." It is rare for this strategy not to occasion a renewal of interest in the underresponsive person. This technique is remarkably effective because the distant person is usually operating automatically, whereas our client, the former pursuer, is operating consciously, with our help.

To complete our glimpse of an Aikido response to conflict when the goal is intimacy, what happens when the intimate partner has become responsive to closeness? Maybe he or she began in a combative mode, but all that excellent listening has softened him or her considerably. Or, perhaps the previously distant person is approaching, or the blamer is now more vulnerable.

Sometimes it gets easy

When there is still a conflict, but the conversation has become calm, it is time to prove the goodwill that one offered during the listening phase. To capitalize on the positive momentum, one can offer to brainstorm a creative solution, as in "I'm glad we're talking about this, and there are clearly valid concerns we both have. Let's put our heads together and see whether we can come up with an option where we'd both be happy."

Of course, intimacy is not always our goal in communication. When the goal is *neutralization*—that is, stopping a verbal attack—the rules change. Once again, we are imagining that the attack has continued despite the careful listening described previously, only now the setting has changed, and so has the goal. We have all had clients, for example, who are being harassed at work, gentle folk who are teased to the point of hidden tears. In selecting an appropriate Aikido strategy, the determining factor is whether the power is equivalent or if one is subordinate. If the power is potentially equal—that is, the attacker is not one's boss or any other type of supervisor—one will still feel intimidated as a recipient of passive-aggressive, sarcastic, or critical behavior. A simple and effective Aikido strategy is *overagreement,* a passive-aggressive retort that draws its power from the attack itself. It removes the power from a verbal assault by extending the very direction of that attack. (Hint: Verbal attacks are literally deflating for people, so remind clients to breathe before responding, or they will run out of air.) Some examples are:

Neutralizing a verbal attack, passive-aggressive version

Attack: "Hey, I'm just kidding—can't you take a joke?"

Defense: "Of course you are. I can always recognize great wit when I see it!"

Attack: "You are a fool."
[Substitute the insult of your choice.]

Defense: "Hey, thanks. I'm so lucky to have such an astute critic to teach me my faults!"

Attack: "Why does it have to be your way all the time?"

Defense: "I guess I never learned to be as flexible and understanding as you."

There is nasty stuff on both sides, but the overagreement is happening in a context in which listening has been offered and the other's intent to control is well demonstrated. Overagreement neutralizes the verbal thrust so easily that there is an all-purpose version that requires no thinking at all. After the insulting comment, an overstated "Right!" pretty much makes the point.

If there is anyone more difficult than passive-aggressive colleagues, it is verbally aggressive colleagues. They yell and challenge, complete with narrowed eyes, knit brows, and thrusting jaws. Sometimes they even have one's boss intimidated in one way or another. There is no point in using force against force with such people. They are usually better at it, having had a lot of practice, and they like it. How can one channel such difficult energy and neutralize it?

Neutralizing aggressive communication

Here are three strategies that fit the bill: First, step outside their universe. Aggressive people are fond of providing a universe of forced choices. They tell you to do something, and this provides you with a decision of complying or not, right? No, there remains an alternative, which is just that: Offer an alternative that works for you. For instance, when people order you around—say, to get you to do their job for them—you might offer to help as soon as you finish something you are already doing, perhaps after making sure it is okay with your boss.

A second strategy is to deflect the attacker's energy through questions. The person asking the questions, as opposed to the person who is in a defensive position, is usually in charge of the conversation. For example, people with offensive communication styles are quick to take offense at innocuous statements, again putting other people on the defense. Questions such as, "Oh, did you think I meant it that way?" or "What gave you that impression?" or "Why would I say that?" all turn the attack back.

For a third approach, especially if the first two are not sufficient to neutralize the trouble, find your trump card. In each setting, there is a set of goals and values that binds everyone. People either believe in these goals or, at least, have to give them lip service. Let's say you are a teacher (perhaps adding the other person's tenure to the difficult mix). Prefacing your suggestion with "Since our mutual goal is the well-being of the children" is likely to align the other person with whatever you say next.

These three strategies are tried and true for situations in which our power is not formally less than the other person's, but is in effect less because of the other person's style. Of course, many other situations find us formally subordinate.

Managing up when reason is of little use

If the power distribution is unequal, one must shy away from techniques such as overagreement. They can be too effective, and others, if they have real power, will exact retribution—because they can. In such a case, an Aikido option is still available, which you might call "pattern making" (as opposed to "pattern breaking"). This is a technique of stimulating automatic patterns in another person to neutralize unfair treatment. Again, we assume that careful listening has been tried or would be of no avail. In other words, a reasonable expectation is that the authority is operating from a rigid and unyielding place. Aikido would suggest that we use this rigid energy, and we will.

Rigid, patterned behavior is predictable and controllable, if we know the right buttons to push. As Virginia Satir and other family systems therapists taught us, dyads contain interlocking parts that create each other. Further, these dyads often reveal parent–child dynamics. "Yes, you can" creates "No, I can't," which in turn creates "Yes, you can." It is the same with "you will" and "I won't." The latter would not be a useful dyad to initiate as a subordinate, would it? On the other hand, "I'm trying hard, please help me" (good kid) creates "I can help you" (helpful parent). Let us see the results of such a pattern-making strategy, illustrated by the following personal story.

I was driving home from my office, fatigued but alert, as I moved toward a left fork through a small town known for vigorous law enforcement. I was driving about nine miles over the speed limit, which police accept in my region. I passed a slower car on the right, which is not acceptable in Connecticut, but I am from New York and get stubborn about that. Noticing that I was passing a police cruiser as I did so, I glanced down to check my speedometer. Satisfied with the results and noticing several speeders passing me, I relaxed. This sense of relief soon passed from me as quickly as the speeding cars. The officer pulled me over, and a wave of confusion spread over me. This feeling would soon prove useful. After the license and registration part, the conversation proceeded.

> "Do you know why I pulled you over, sir?"
>
> "No, officer, I'm wondering."
>
> "You were driving 58 miles per hour in a 40-mile zone, and passing on the right, weaving through traffic."

I felt startled. I knew the part about the speed was untrue. In fact, I knew this with a certainty only surpassed by the fact that denying it would be useless. I continued, listening carefully. "I was going 58?" Note that I was focusing on the one part of the accusation I was certain was untrue. I knew that the radar must have hit another auto. Perhaps he wondered also.

"Yes, sir, you were," was his answer. "We are keeping a close eye on things. You know, with the road rage problem."

"Wow. I knew I was tired, but I didn't think I was that tired. I'm glad you stopped me."

"You're glad?"

"I'm careful not to speed. If I was going anything like that speed, I clearly didn't know what I was doing. You might have saved my life."

"Why do you say that?"

"I can't be driving like that, tired or not. I was sure I was driving safely, but I'm hearing that I was wrong."

"Listen, I'm just going to give you a verbal warning this time."

"Whatever you think is right."

"Most people that I stop, they have terrible attitudes. You seem to get the point."

"They don't know what you're doing out here."

"Have a good day, sir."

Of course, this is not meant as a primer on avoiding traffic tickets. The fact is that I believed that the outcome I sought was just, and I meant every word I said. The only way for me to have been speeding would be if I were hallucinating a different speedometer. I went with his reality, a cooperative "kid," so he could be a helpful "parent" (although I was significantly older than he was).

In this way, intentional use of patterns can neutralize conflict. It is even possible to use parental behavior with a boss, as long as it is distant-critical behavior, not angry-correcting behavior. Asking pointed questions to pin down a criticism would fit this technique. We can experiment and role-play to find effective responses and help our clients practice them. The client will recognize, as we will, which type of response produces a neutralizing effect on the difficult person in his or her life.

Finally, when the goal of communication is enrollment, securing cooperation from a less-than-cooperative person, one asks oneself a different follow-up question during the assessment phase: Do we have the leverage of any common interest? If so, we have access to a powerful form of Aikido, *matching motivations*. For example, if I am a psychological consultant who wants to market team-building strategies to a corporation, my pitch that these strategies will humanize the workplace is probably less effective than a demonstration that my consulting techniques will improve corporate profits.

How to enroll cooperation

Everyone has a set of priorities, often both unstated and unaware. Yet these unstated values identify themselves when we observe the choices that people make. Most of us would agree that helping other people, having the esteem of others, being financially successful, performing at one's peak, and excelling in one's field are worthy endeavors. However, in which order would you place these? Or are there other values that you would prize more highly, such as seeking spiritual growth, winning the love of others, establishing security, or finding sensory enjoyment? When one of us wants an outcome, we want it because it seems very good to us in terms of our own values.

Since people's priorities vary, effective salespeople learn this, and they will ask you questions before they suggest any benefit to their products. Some potential customers want control, others want an impressive image, others want precision, and others want support. Successful salespeople will frame their product's benefits in terms of their take on which of these is paramount to a potential customer. Similarly, if you look to mobilize support by appealing to a benefit that does not interest the other person, you will either put that person to sleep or annoy him or her.

Approaching this sequentially, one can begin by defining one's own objective in any situation. Second, one discerns the motivating factors for the other person whom you want to enroll. The clues to this motivation are found by watching how the other person makes decisions and which directions he or she typically pursues. Finally, drawing a figurative straight line, one can look for the manner in which one's objective could match the other's motivation.

This works because there can be several possible benefits to a desired course of action. Using a business example, will it improve the quality of life for coworkers, improve the bottom line financially, enhance the reputation of the department, or ease the workload on management? Rather than speaking in terms of which of these benefits most appeals to you, instead you would speak about whichever of them seems most likely to appeal to the decision maker. When you apply such a line of reasoning, you will have your audience's attention, if not their immediate cooperation.

Finally, we turn to the difficult circumstance in which you must mobilize support but can find no positive motivation to use for leverage.

Getting something with nothing

The operative words here, "must" and "no," in combination, present an important challenge. The situation is important, but there is no known bond of interest. Rather than having the lack of a common motivational link signal defeat, one can ask a different question: If you and the person lack a common interest, is there perhaps something that this other person does not want to happen, some outcome they would find adverse? It might seem that this line of reasoning is leading toward our making a threat, but such an action would not be a Aikido approach.

In fact, if one threatens applying a strong force at another, it often inspires greater force back. For this reason, research on the effects of fear-arousing public health appeals confused social psychologists because of conflicting results of the studies. Meta-analyses finally revealed that fear increased persuasion to a point, but then reversed its effect if the fear became too provocative. That is why smoking cessation programs so often fail. One might call this the "cornered squirrel" effect: Back people into a corner, and they have nothing to lose by striking back at you. Much more effective, because it aligns mutual interest in avoiding a future threat, is a mild fear-provoking response, such as a "non-threat."

What is a non-threat? This technique subtly implies a threat by proposing a mutual attempt to avoid it. Instead of daring the other person, "If you don't cooperate in this endeavor, I will bring legal action!" a non-threat gently suggests, "I really want to work this out. I'm trying hard to handle this *in*formally with you." The emphasis on the prefix "in" can be essential. It makes the point of proffered cooperation. Yet, the very same emphasis simultaneously sets off the word "formally" as an implication and a possible future step. With no overt threat, the non-threat urges the other person to be responsible while it is his or her free choice.

If stated collegially, a non-threat can suggest that both parties jointly want to take some course of action because they both do not want to have the future exposure of having failed to act. In this case, one actually enters a protector role, heading off danger for the other. Of course, there is clearly some pressure implicit to voicing such a warning.

This is a powerful strategy, and it is appropriate to use only sparingly, perhaps rarely. Effective though the non-threat is, it clearly does not encourage future goodwill with the difficult other party. On the other hand, *respect* is a different matter. Whether or not your client applies this strategy, the knowledge of it creates a sense of personal power. It illustrates Aikido's effects even during the challenging test of complacent disregard by another.

The essential point to keep in mind about Aikido is that whatever works best tends to work this way. As a result, we could create an ever-expanding list of applications of synchronized momentum to almost any endeavor we would explore. Although such Tao-inspired strategies are remarkable, the key to applying Aikido is to understand it as a frame of mind. Most of them resulted by my maintaining an Aikido attitude, while identifying with the interpersonal dilemmas posed to me by people in therapy sessions. With a similar stance, you will generate your own strategies. Keeping that in focus, we will next notice a surprising application of this phenomenon to the management of rigid patterns of behavior, and then we will look closely at client resistance.

There are endless applications of Aikido to psychotherapy

The Stress-Regress: The Hinge on Which Freedom Rotates

Of all the Aikido magic that one can work in sessions, there is one dimension of the human condition that seems to stand out from all the rest: the obvious but elusive fact that people regress to rigid behavior patterns during high stress. This phenomenon is a commonsense observation, to the point that few people would deny that our actions seem to become more automatic under excessive pressure. Managing this stress-regress is elusive just the same, though, because of its effects. Reduced awareness during high stress guarantees that people will tend not to notice the switch into automatic behavior, at least in themselves.

This is important. It is awfully discouraging for people to discover that they cannot use what they learn, including in your psychotherapy sessions, when they most need it. Stress is a function of how important some event is to us. Therefore, if the pressure is getting high, so are our stakes in the outcomes. Close relationships, important interviews, attempts to change personality, efforts to break out of our "erroneous zones"—if it matters, it is important enough to make it likely that we will forget whatever we have learned when we try to deal with it. This is also what prevents most self-help books from being very helpful.

Why people lose therapeutic insights when they need them most

You now know the reason that our clients (and we) often cannot recall, let alone apply, the insights of therapy when it most counts. When the brain moves into automatic responses, it will select them based on factors such as practice and familiarity—hence the regression. Not preparing ourselves and our clients for this is one of the main reasons that many people do not believe that anyone can change and therefore see little value in therapy.

Although the subject is unaware of the move into predictable, automatic patterns during the stress-regress and it seems unpredictable and erratic to others, researchers can see it imaged in the brain. We will return to this when we review methods to integrate Aikido strategies into existing theories. For now, our point is that this is a universal, inevitable phenomenon. This also makes good biological sense, which is why it comes with the original equipment. Part of the way that our complex and deep-thinking brains stay in Tao harmony with the environment is through switching into a rapid-response mode during physical emergencies. The price for this excellent adaptation to the immediacy of danger is that our brains do the same thing in any perceived danger, including interpersonal stress. During social demands, however, the ability to flexibly choose, or even invent, behavior would be better. That is where we come in handy as therapists.

Being attentive to the stress-regress offers two main advantages to psychotherapy practice. First, we can prepare our clients for the fact that this is going to happen; second, we can plan to make new learning available when it is most needed. Let us say, for example, that you have taught someone one of the communication strategies discussed previously. You are both pleased at the expectation that this could make a distressing situation work better. This is a nice thought—but it probably will not happen, at least not yet. Here are the kinds of instructions you might provide to make these strategies available during stress:

Managing the stress-regress

> I'm glad that you think this could work, and I think it can too. Now we have to make it available when you need it, when it's stressful. The thing about stress is that we become much more automatic, and the same old patterns come up every time. So the best way to access this new skill when you need it is to leave it where you'll be able to find it. We have to attach it right onto the old pattern. What would work is to practice it until it gets more familiar. Then, imagine past times that you would have wanted to use it and practice moving from the problem into the solution. If you do this a bunch of times, you will start to connect the problem with

the way out of it. You can then imagine future situations that haven't happened yet, again practicing doing this.

You can see the practical power this can add to our strategies. Essentially, we are adding an extra step between the two elements of change that therapists already supply. We know well the importance of providing new insights into a problem area, and we recognize the value of developing alternative ways to respond. Connecting these two, we want to offer pattern interrupters to break the rigidity. This might consist of chaining the alternative, with practice, onto the old response, as modeled here. Alternatively, it might include chaining any methods that short-circuit the old behavior pattern directly onto the old pattern itself. The best of these pattern-breaking methods will typically retrieve content filtered out by the automatic response, such as incompatible information or feelings.

Three steps to reliable change

For example, the many slogans of Alcoholics Anonymous are repeated often in meetings in the hope that the important pattern-breaking insight, such as "It's the first drink that does it," are chained onto the urge to rationalize taking a drink. Our previously suggested strategy of using the wrong feeling to find the right one would also benefit from such pattern-breaking practice. One could practice moving from the depression cover-up to the underlying anger or from an anger cover-up to the underlying sadness, depending on the person. As happily useful as these kinds of augmentations to therapy are, probably the most uniquely instrumental application of the stress-regresss insight is in the area of increasing self-esteem.

Whether stated or not, the most deeply haunting question in many therapy sessions is, "How could I?" In other words, what is

How making peace with the stress-regress helps self-esteem

the matter with me that I keep making the same mistake? Even psychological models can reinforce this, whether developmental (such as humanistic or psychoanalytic) models or aggregate learning (such as behaviorist or cognitive–behaviorist) models. Both our culture and our theories can lead to people judging themselves by their worst moments.

On the other hand, most of our clients do not have personality disorders, and they can compare the parts of their lives that work well with the parts that seldom do. The good news is that we can leverage their successful areas, tapping into strengths that can be brought into the problem areas. Without a better way to frame this disparity, however, these areas of error can lead to embarrassment and shame.

This challenge is managed well by a discussion of the stress-regress. As you will note, one of the joys of practical Aikido insights, such as synchronizing self-esteem with the stress-regress, is that we can understand them without becoming abstract and theoretical. Two examples of such a conversation about this phenomenon could be called "instant analysis" and the "worst thing you can say about yourself." Let us sample a couple of scripts for such a presentation.

First, the instant analysis:

> You wonder why you do this, and I can show you how to do an instant analysis of any rigid habit. It goes like this:
>
> - You do it now because you did it before.
> - You did it before because you learned it.
> - You learned it because it worked for you or someone at that time.

Though simple, this is an accurate vision of the picture we get when we look through the lens of insight into the stress-regress. Further, it directly leads us into the next point:

> When people first come to see me, they sometimes think that they are problematic people. As we explore and understand the situation better, they no longer think that they *are* the problem, but that they *have* a problem. Later, they come to see that this problem is just an old behavior pattern, so that now they have a pattern. Finally, they realize that this pattern is just an old, outdated skill. The fact that it is outdated is actually a good sign—it means that you have succeeded in living in a different setting than the one you learned it in. Otherwise, it would still fit. So if you want to give yourself a hard time, you can say anything, but if you want to be accurate, the worst thing you can say about yourself is that some of your old patterns are outdated.

Over the years, a few illuminating metaphors for this have emerged from sessions. One is the ice skating rink, in which I suggested, "If you had grown up on an ice-skating rink, whenever it was really important to get somewhere in a hurry, you'd move like this," whereupon I stand up and mimic trying to skate across the carpet, meeting much more resistance than walking would encounter.

Handy stress-regress metaphors

This metaphor is dramatic for its visual effects, whereas the power of the next one amply compensates for needing to rely on one's imagination. It consists of a story:

> Imagine that your childhood was like having to walk through a forest. Your biggest problem is that many people

> are throwing stones at you. Not only do these stones hurt a lot, but they could destroy you. So you duck behind a tree, but this is no solution. Your task is to make your way to the lake. But you are resourceful, and you discover that you can strip the bark off the tree, and you use the vines growing on it to make armor for yourself. You start out and it really works! The stones still come, but they don't hurt as much, and none does you harm. Sure enough, you make it to the lake. As you enter the lake, things get better because you now can duck under the water and elude your attackers, adding a great new option. So you head out across the lake. All is well at first, but then disaster strikes. You find that you can't swim because something is dragging you down. What is it? It is the very same armor that saved you before. It is becoming waterlogged. *Exactly what protected you before is now hurting you in situations of threat.* We have to learn to untie it and free you.

These are all delightful conversations to have with someone, as is typical of the pleasures of operating from synchronized momentum. Aikido is why the stress-regress strategies are so helpful, as they put us in synchronized harmony with our own nature. Putting the matter another way, these strategies are just a case of Aikido applied in alignment with the force of the stress-regress.

How to Make Resistance Work for You

As we move to the next application, client resistance to treatment, the first point to keep in mind is that your encountering defensiveness or resistance may sometimes mean that you are coming across as judgmental. When you operate with a peer attitude and an Aikido frame of mind, your clients will usually tell you that they feel comfortable with you, especially when this was not the case in previous counseling they have done. Even so, we all hit walls at times.

Being a therapist means coaching people when they are somehow stuck in their lives. They may remain so even after they work with us. We may blame ourselves for delayed progress, and some clients may help us assign the blame to ourselves. Of course, they may even be correct, if we have failed to develop an attitude of alliance, or if we leave the development of effective change techniques to our clients. Other times, especially for the sort of therapist who would be drawn to a text such as this, the fault may be neither our clients' nor ours. The client has simply hit a barrier, one that he or she does not yet understand.

Joke: How many therapists does it take to change a light bulb? Just one, but only if the light bulb really wants to change.

Of course, all who seek therapy really want to change, at least theoretically. In practice, though, our clients' entire worlds change when they do, because every rebirth requires a death of that which came before. Furthermore, some of the friends and family in their lives may be hindering change because of the same fears. So the experience of recoil is natural, but the frame in which we place this experience will tend to determine its future. The following therapeutic metaphor synchronizes therapy momentum with the temporary experience of a barrier, so that it bodes progress rather than failure, when people report being stuck:

Ch-ch-ch-changes

> After I know where you want to go, I always begin by drawing the shortest distance between two points on that road. Then I access all the strategies I have ever learned, and suggest the most direct path. Afterward, you leave the session, and one of two things happens. You either get there easily, in which case we celebrate, or you hit a pothole and don't arrive where

> you thought you were going. That's no problem. It just tells us that a hindrance has come up from your past learning to stop you. Now we know where to dig, to uncover what came up, and learn how to get past it. Rather than digging up the whole road, we keep our focus on the present and glance back to the past when necessary.

Sometimes, one can go more in-depth, as follows.

> This is the difference between counseling and therapy. Counseling is a strategic process. It is the search for steps toward change, using broader thinking, developing new skills, or finding useful old skills. If you hit a barrier when you try to take these steps, therapy glances back to the past to uncover the source of these barriers and clear them up. The barriers can be very old habits or beliefs that become rigid during stressful times. Then, ways to move past these barriers can be designed. In this way, counseling and therapy work together.

Most people get this immediately, and it accurately frames the experience of being stuck as the signal to learn something new. Neutralizing resistance by reframing it, we thus transmute resistance into an opportunity. This actually puts us in reach, as we will next explore, of gaining benefits from what is otherwise the greatest hindrance to psychotherapeutic success.

An Example of Using Resistance: First-Thought Questions

One specific technique that directly harnesses the energy of resistance to make change happen is the first-thought question. Let us look at how this plays out with what looks like a total block of communication. This is a second session with a man who is very apprehensive about where I might take him. In our first visit, we mostly talked about talking, about what therapy and counseling are. I framed it as a form of coaching, and now he is willing to concede that it is worth checking out. We do not have an alliance yet, as the following conversation shows. Again, my comments are in italics. Note that the "it" he is not ready to describe can remain just an "it."

"I don't want to talk about it!"

Then let's agree that we are not going to talk about it. In fact, rather than talking about it, let's talk about not talking about it.

"What does that mean? Isn't that the same?"

That's not what I have in mind. I'm really looking to explore how important it is for you not to talk about this, so we can learn some new things without getting into the subject.

"How could that work?"

Well, I'm going to ask you only to repeat things you are already saying, so we can both really hear them. I will ask you questions, but only about what you are already saying, not new information.

"Maybe you have to show me."

Exactly. So, here's just one suggestion: Say the first thing that comes into your mind without trying to make sense of it. Then, we can make sense of it later.

"Okay."

So, tell me again that you don't want to talk about it.

"I don't."

You don't what?

"I don't want to talk about it."

Good. Again.

"I don't want to talk about it, and I'm not going to."

Exactly. One more time.

"I don't want to talk about it."

What happens if you do—first thought?

"Nothing."

Again.

"Nothing happens."

Good. And what does nothing feel like—first thought?

"Nothing doesn't feel—it's just nothing."

When do you feel nothing?

"Most of the time, I mean, I don't know what I'm feeling most of the time, so it's pretty much nothing to me."

And what's it like there?

"Like nothing. There's no 'there.'"

So, it's nowhere.

"Kind of."

So, it's like nowhere. Can you repeat that?

"It's like nothing, nowhere."

Where do you want to be—first thought?

"Not nowhere."

And you know that.

"That, I know."

That's a start.

We have just aligned for the first time, agreeing that moving from the emptiness, from the numb place in which he lives, is our common goal. His resistance thus provides the energy to go deeper, as we apply the exact moment of reticence as a thrust to move forward. We rely on the signs of hesitation to cue our probe. In this case, I did not want to explain too much, but I will often elaborate, as I begin first-thought inquiries, especially if the person hesitates:

The deeper the resistance, the greater the energy

Your first thoughts may be things you don't believe. We're looking to learn what the automatic pattern is telling you, not what your real beliefs today are telling you. We'll make sense out of it later.

This frees your client's verbalizations so the patterned thoughts spontaneously arise. The following are some additional tips in developing this strategy:

- ☯ A good time to apply first-thought questions is when clients make global decisions, especially those of the "I can't," "I won't," "it's never," or "it's always" varieties. Chronic distress—for example, discouragement or fear—is another signal to try this. It is also a nice technique for those times a client reports a big disparity between the wishes of the mind and the dictates of the heart.
- ☯ We are looking for connections, not logic. The unconscious processes work by sequences and associations, not by reason.
- ☯ A typical format would be for the client to repeat the generalized thought several times. This both intensifies the experience and detaches the idea from its rationalizations.

- Next, say the first-thought question quickly, enhancing the element of surprise. The questions, such as "What happens if you do?" "What might happen next?" "Who says so?" or "Like when?" are prompting the next connection in the sequence. Often, you will complete the question with "first thought," such as "What happens if you do? First thought!"
- You can follow up the answer, either by having that be the next repeated statement, or asking one of the above questions, or a new one, such as "And what then?" "What's the worst that might happen?" "Until what?" "How can you tell? or "What would you like?"
- If the individual hesitates to answer, you might prompt spontaneity by directing "That one!" meaning "Voice the thought that just went fleeting by." If the person says her or his mind is blank, respond with Aikido and suggest, "Say 'blank.'" Then, go back to the repetitions.

How We Can Use Pain from the Past to Free Up the Present

Another way that people can be stuck is inside feelings of association between a bad memory and a new situation. We may be well aware that the emotional connection is bogus. In fact, this might be the crux of our frustration. It seems so "stupid" to be bound up in the feelings that we had for a situation that is over, even as we are preparing for a new experience. This false identification can occur regarding people as well. Then, it seems even quirkier, as we can often see that our emotional reactions are inappropriate.

As we apply an Aikido filter of synchronized momentum, it becomes clear that it is necessary to accept the association before we try to break it. We cannot break a rigid response pattern if we do not allow ourselves to have it. Because the association is painful, we all naturally prefer to focus only on all the ways in which the two situations are different. This will work only if the association is very weak. However, if that were going to work in this case, it would have already done so, and you would not have heard about it from your client. Knowing that the association is rigid, we go with it.

I first heard about this technique as an "identity check" from practitioners of "co-counseling," a mutual counseling strategy in which rapidly dispatching false associations between people is frequently necessary. The instructions that I use for this strategy are specific and fully portable for homework practice.

- ☯ Note every single similarity you can between the two situations, no matter how trivial a comparison. Don't stop until you cannot come up with a single additional point of comparison.
- ☯ After noticing all the similarities, validate how it is makes sense that you would have associated the two experiences.
- ☯ Now that you are truly done making the connection, note every single difference you can between the two experiences. Again, include even little points of contrast.
- ☯ Write this down to recreate the experience and reinforce it. As simple as this is, it has a powerful effect, fueled by the power of harnessing the negative association itself.

The Tao Wisdom and Method of Making Friends with One's Childhood

An old "sick" joke (I think it was by comedian Tommy Smothers, circa 1962) went something like: "You know, I have the heart of a small boy. Yes, I keep it right in my drawer." Those were more innocent times, during which it was widely inconceivable that anyone would actually mortally harm a small child. Geographically, of course you do not have an inner child. You cannot find one either in your drawer or in your elbow. Neither can your clients. In terms of memory, we would not expect to find a discrete inner-child entity. Every age that we ever have been should comprise a continuum of recollection, with significant events indelibly etched in memory. Thus, childhood memory would seem to be a range of recall, rather than any duality.

Psychologically, though, the "inner child" is an apt metaphor because of the nature of emotional defenses. The best established of these defenses is our capacity for denial of painful memories. Denial keeps the unthinkable comfortably unknowable for a while. We exile painful reminiscences from consciousness, because we can. As a result, it is as if we have a hurting inner "self." Paradoxically, this "old" version of oneself is, of course, very young. Eventually, we need to return to these childhood memories to achieve freedom. For example, important information is hiding within the child.

The basis and nature of the old, young self

Naturally, while we were hurting, we were also making some imperative decisions: who we must be; who we cannot be; what we cannot do; what we must do. These directives, unconsidered, become the premises of our future decisions. Although these limitations eventually confined us, we originally created them to best survive during excruciating moments of childhood. They worked best then, which is why we did them, and here we are. Now that we are adults, these premises no longer accurately define our parameters. These childhood confinements send us messages such as:

- You have nothing useful to say.
- No one will love you for yourself.

- Love means staying close to people who hurt you.
- No one will care about what you want unless you scare them.
- You are ultimately a disappointment.

Once we have achieved renewed access to the cache of these unwelcome experiences, inside that box of pain, we have new choices about the premises we had established. We can reconsider and edit them.

Achieving this requires going with the sensed presence of an inner child, even the most painful parts of that childhood experience. Inner-child work, when useful, establishes ongoing communication. In contrast, "healing your inner child" workshops are often resolution-oriented and tend to have a single, common flaw: They often promote completion. This, in effect, attempts to exile the hurting child again; we aim to be done with him or her.

How many clients, having had previous therapy, have said to you that there is no need to get into it? "We don't have to work on that part, because I already did it. I worked it through with my previous therapist." Of course, if that were true, they would not trouble themselves with leading you off the trail. Their communication would be more in the manner of, "That part of me is something I'm acquainted with from my last counselor. I don't know if there is any more to learn about it."

In contrast to final resolution, *the point of inner-child work is to establish an ongoing link for communication and friendly rapport.* This pushed-away part of us thinks we want to kill it, because we have often tried to do so. We do not want to experience its pain, but this attempt to excise the past has been unfair of us. The congealed box of memories is not intending to hurt us; it is simply in pain and has no one, including us,

Adopting one's own early self

to protect it. It cannot go away because it is real, if only a recording. Not only can it be brought into communication, but it will also actually make deals with us that are of mutual benefit. In truth, there are no inner enemies. We see this type of progress in the following vignette.

Ronnie arrives at the office, anxious about ever finding a relationship. This pattern, in the past, has guaranteed rapidly and poorly chosen partners. Warning signs were regularly overlooked. Friends had counseled that "you have to be okay alone before you are ready for a good relationship," but it was easier said than done. This is our fifth session. Ronnie has some insight about the past, and may be ready to apply it.

> "I know that worrying about it doesn't help. It actually turns off people I date sometimes. So I hide it. But, it's what I do, whether it helps or not."
>
> *Did it ever help?*
>
> "With finding a good relationship?"
>
> *With anything.*
>
> "Well, my mother likes me that way, you know. Her motto is 'the family that worries together stays together' (laughs), but I can't say it worked too well."
>
> *So, is there a part of you suggesting this as a useful approach to getting close?*
>
> "Yeah, I guess you could say that I would have learned that love is worrying with people. So, you think that I'm telling myself to worry so that I can find someone to love?"
>
> *Sounds like it could fit. What's your sense?*
>
> "Oh, it fits the past great. Doesn't help me much now, though."

Well, what does this early part of you actually want?

"It just wants love, you know, closeness."

Maybe we could work a deal.

"Like, what?"

What deal would you like to have with this small, lonely, worried part of you?

"If I could get cooperation?

(*Nod*)

"Oh. Well, I would agree to bring around lots of friends, if the little-kid-me would only let me be myself."

Offer that deal, that if you are free to feel confident, you'll supply good company, and see how that feels inside. Keep in mind that this part of you is not accustomed to your talking to it, so it may be wary.

(*After twenty seconds*) "Actually, I feel strange. Like a nice, settling feeling, as if that deal really happened. Can it happen like that?"

Well, I'll tell you, I've felt things like that, so it makes sense to me. Remind yourself a few times each day about this deal, and see if it continues to feel right.

Using force against force, we either want to destroy these painful memories, or digest the little kid, absorbing it forever. Harmonizing energy, we start to hang out, protect, and learn from the little person we once were, and we begin to like that child. The child has gifts to give back to us: an open heart, play, and the freedom to drive our lives where we want to, rather than having a little boy or girl at the wheel. Without the inner kid, who comes equipped with the well-preserved experience of being a child, we would not so well remember how it felt to kid around!

The Aikido of Medication

In this section on psychotherapeutic strategies, we should also look at the question of whether medication is consistent with the Tao of your psychotherapy practice. It may seem that the least Aikido-ish thing to do with our feelings is to medicate them. After all, emotional pain provides both the signal and the motivation to change our lives. There is also no doubt that the least brilliant psychiatrists have been prone to reduce all psychological issues to "chemical imbalances," although I have never seen a study in the research literature that draws such a conclusion.

Then again, there are also many awful psychotherapists. (We can talk about them freely, as they have stopped reading by now.) Similarly, the best psychiatrists (according to one of them, Dr. Irene Abramovich in the Hartford, CT area), encourage therapy, recognizing that the meds stop working if the emotional and cognitive patterns remain unchanged. So, what do the best psychiatrists offer us as therapists? For people who are too overwhelmed by their current symptoms to apply what you are working on together, medications turn down the volume on suffering. As a result, there is indeed an Aikido of medication.

We can think of the stuck areas of our lives as being trapped down in the pit, and we often do. Therapy teaches someone how to climb out and even throws a useful rope down. This is fine when an individual feels up to climbing. On the other hand, if all that time down the pit has atrophied the psychological muscles and softened the

Lessons of the pit

cognitive hands, all that rope can supply are rope burns as one falls back down. How about pills alone? That is kind of like throwing some drugs down into the pit and saying, "Hey, you might be happier down there with these." Therapy and medication together (again, when the current pain is too distracting to focus on anything else) is like rolling down a rope ladder. With concentration and a good grip, most people can climb it.

This reminds me of taking Nyquil® when I have a cold. I know I have to rest, but if the symptoms are strong, sleep is elusive. The symptomatic relief does not cure the cold, but it makes it easier for me to cure it myself. In this way, it is good to let people who are having particularly tough times know about the medication options, especially in light of recent medication improvements. When someone elects to use meds, be sure to use explanatory metaphors, such as the Nyquil one, so they still give themselves credit for making the changes that ultimately are the only way out of the pit.

In addition, there seem to be people who do have organically driven mood issues. Even after dealing effectively with cognitive, emotional, interpersonal, behavioral, and spiritual patterns, you get an "organic feel" that suggests that a person's body is working against him or her. Here again, medication is a way of working with, rather than against, the presentation.

Having expressed this, I admit that I still prefer avoiding medications most of the time. Both the motivation for change and the signs of progress come from psychological pain; it is my ally as a therapist. However, as we can see, there is a way that medication is helpful as well as the way that experienced pain is helpful. Our job is to seek a harmonized balance.

3

How to Provide Escape from the Pendulum of Rigid Mindsets

Double-Stuck: The Dichotomous Story of "Pendulemia"

We have already noted that one of the useful Aikido strategies is that of sharing information on the stress–regress. I also refer to the stress–regress as "state-rigidity," as it is a state of cognitive rigidity and automatic behavior triggered by high stress. This information has a powerful effect on helping retrieve self-esteem for your most earnest clients, those who do not shirk awareness of their shortcomings. Making people aware of the stress–regress also allows specific techniques to anticipate and correct for it.

Probably nothing we will explore in this text is more important than this. *If we do not anticipate and correct for state-rigidity, our sessions will be about as useful as the typical self-help book.* People read and agree, get excited, but soon fail to apply the new insights when they are most needed. Thus, of all the phenomena in need of Aikido grace, state-rigidity is among the most crucial for change.

What does high stress shift do to the mind? It confines perception to a narrow track, splits thinking into either–or extremes, and makes responses automatic. Because they are selected automatically (by the amygdala; see LeDoux, 1998), responses must be already learned, and the oldest patterns tend to be the best learned. This explains the regressive nature of these automatic behaviors. (For many references on this phenomenon, see the bibliography at the end of this book.) Because flexible thought and responses become filtered out, this change results in, and is maintained, by a temporary state of rigidity.

Now, let us look at how to be useful about this. One can intervene in any of these rigid areas—the thinking, perception, or habits—but there is a distinct advantage to the thinking element: this is the most conscious aspect of this largely unconscious state. Even when people are stressed out, they can usually count to two. So, if I am able to come up with only two responses to a dilemma, both of them unpleasant, this tells me that I am likely in the state of rigidity. Mr. Spock was right when he advised Captain Kirk (on the original Star Trek series), "There are always alternatives, Captain." The Spock character, the show's voice of reason, was urging his commander to look beyond extreme and dichotomous reactions during an emergency. The literature also agrees that dichotomous thinking is one of the typical results of stressful cognition (Meichenbaum 1977).

Awareness of state-rigidity consciousness is itself a type of Aikido technique. We are now going to expand this into "pendulemia" strategies. *Pendulemia* is a catchy name, useful for clients, to refer to this type of cognitive state-rigidity, as the mind swings between two choices—I often call them "awful" and "terrible." Of course, it affects us as much as it affects our clients.

Although we will explore practice strategies in depth later, our current discussion of pendulemia is an opportunity too great to miss, as we begin to see how our own thinking can become dichotomous in our work as psychotherapists. So, let us digress to that subject briefly.

What to Do When 'Pendulemia' Attacks Your Practice

"Black and white," "either–or," or dichotomous choices are endemic to stress thinking. As pressure rises, gray areas recede, and awareness becomes captured by falsely polarized opposites. This holds true for our clients; it is equally so for their therapists. The age of managed care has been nothing if not stressful for us as psychotherapists. Thus, our choices often seem falsely confined to dichotomies.

- ☯ Will we be employed or work for ourselves?
- ☯ Will we provide long-term treatment for a few wealthy clients, or symptom-oriented brief therapy that is affordable to many?
- ☯ Do we join managed care panels against our wishes, or do we firmly refuse even to send outpatient treatment reports (OTRs) for our clients?
- ☯ Do we seek the security of working in approved group practices, or do we settle for the lower income of a part-time but private practice?

Learning to use the forces working against us to our advantage will require our moving beyond these false choices. For example, offering a monthly treatment option, when appropriate, breaks out of the dichotomy between joining HMOs and having a part-time practice. (We will expand on this option in the next chapter.) As we will see, beginning within the security of employment, we can begin an intermittent therapy practice. With enough finesse, we could provide effective long-term treatment that is affordable to many. We can thus stay out of panels, sending in OTRs as necessary, but as out-of-plan providers. Using this approach and without joining a group practice, we can build up a full-fee full-time practice. This plan will receive a more detailed description in the chapter on practice structure, but we can already see that it is not confined to the forced choices within which many of us have learned to operate.

So, we and our clients have the same condition—the human condition—in which false dichotomies capture awareness during stress.

This "pendulemia" is at the root of the dichotomous thinking that has therapists losing the war for private practice before firing a shot. Most errors of judgment have their cause in pendulemia, including our own expectations of clinical practice. In both cases, marvelous wizardry lies between the black and white distinctions.

Correcting the Greatest Cause of Bad Judgment

The following therapy session occurred in 1981. In those early days, "What has brought you to see me?" was a frequent first question for me, so that is how I started this session, with the wife of a prominent physician and civic leader in her town. Janice had a prim and reserved quality in both her hairstyle and facial style of expression. Her eyes, however, blazed quietly with some kind of power not fully in her control, and her wit showed a spirit that perhaps needed less control. I soon learned about both.

> "I'm here because I eat my husband for dinner every evening."
>
> *That's an interesting expression.*
>
> "It's true; just ask my kids."
>
> *What happens?*
>
> "I begin the meal civilized enough, put out the food, joining the family just like a normal person. Only, by the end, I am screaming at Doug, and he is asking whether I am all right. Of course I'm not all right. I just lost my mind. Actually, my getting this counseling was his idea before mine. But, I'm quite unhappy about it—the situation, I mean, not the counseling."
>
> *Sounds like quite a mystery. I have to say, you don't look insane*

to me. Maybe we could find out some more details about what happens before you become upset. What goes on in your home in the evening?

"Not much. I'm with the children. Doug comes home and does his normal routine. I fix dinner. They try to eat. I devour Doug. That's it."

What's his normal routine?

"Also not too unusual. He has a stiff martini or two. He makes a call or two. He probably prays about dinner, but I would be guessing."

Whom does he call? Before the possible praying, I mean.

"He calls his girlfriend. (*no change in expression*) I shouldn't call her that. She's much older. Maybe she's more his mother. She's actually a former patient and a political ally, and they talk about whatever. Then he comes down and asks me about what I haven't gotten done today. There you go, a normal day."

How do you react during all this?

"I don't. I've learned that my reactions, so to speak, are not appropriate or helpful. I try to keep myself from acting up, and I usually can behave myself for a while. Then, I blow it."

(A few moments of silence go by, as I imagine an invisible pendulum swinging back and forth.)

You know, I think I might know what's going on.

"That makes one of us."

Let me run it by you. But, I warn you, it's a bit different from your view of yourself.

"How different?"

Well, I think you might be too nice (quizzical expression back). *Surprised?*

"I would be if I believed you."

Well, let me run it by you. You view yourself as an angry, inappropriate person. You distrust your responses and try to stifle them. Meanwhile, your husband comes home every night and proceeds to anger you. He might even know about that; I can't tell. The feeling builds up and builds up, until you lose tolerance, and boom! Once again, you are the cause of all the problems of the family, so you try again to keep yourself in check. Make sense?

"I can't argue with the sequence. But, I still shouldn't blow up."

Actually, I agree. It makes you the problem, and you lose credibility. But how about this: if you spoke up sooner, while it's smaller, you'd start to make sense. Either Doug would start to hear your point of view on some things, or at the least you would see your own point of view. So, it would be win–win.

"I'd try it, if you can show me a better way to get my point across."

Of course I could, as any reader of this text also could. First, I needed to see and to show my client that she was thinking in extreme opposites. In the years since 1981, when Janice first visited me and discovered that she was not a monster, I have often glimpsed such a polarization of choices.

The phenomenon consists of a rigid dichotomy of choices, like a cognitive pendulum, hence the term "pendulemia." There seem to be two varieties. Janice's type, in which the individual cycles back and forth between dual extremes, could be called "cycling pendulemia." (As in bipolar disorder, we can find

Would you like to swing on a star?

both rapid cycling and relatively static versions of cycling pendulemia.) Another variety, in which people spend their whole lives on one opposing polarity in order to stay as far away as possible from the other, can be termed "frozen pendulemia."

Here is a nervy claim: most errors of judgment that humans make consist of some version of pendulemia. Take politics (please). Perhaps you have heard the expression, "A conservative is a liberal who has been mugged." There is also a counterpart, which is, "A liberal is a conservative who has been arrested." This humorously illustrates a process of choosing one polarized opposite in reaction against the other pole. Similarly, political arguments in favor of one point of view are often fallaciously persuasive when they use the "slippery slope" argument about the other side. Presenting one extreme point of view provides motivation to adopt the opposite point of view. This is sometimes also called a "straw man" argument, because it sets up a ridiculous extreme of an opposing argument, so that it can be knocked down as easily as a straw man.

One need go no further than any setting in which there are children and parents to see another common example of pendulemia. Permissive and authoritarian parents both present the other as justification for their own mistakes. "Do it now or else!" and "Please, honey, don't pour your milk on Uncle James's head" both stare at each other, each frozen in position on opposite sides of the room. As costly as each of these mistakes is for all concerned, and as confused as the parents may become, they tend to remain convicted by their revulsion of the opposite point of view. A glance at other parents—perhaps at their own parents—making the opposite type of mistake quickly quells any doubts they might otherwise have about their parenting style.

Pendulemic impossibilities

In the United States, we can watch a sociological case study in pendulemia between the late 1960s and early 1970s. One hears a joking suggestion that if you remember the '60s counterculture, then you obviously were not there. Though cute, this is untrue. Sixties drug use, like sixties promiscuity, was inaccurately perceived. The prevalences of drugs and sex were both exaggerated, both by the older generation of that time and by later, sentimental baby boomers. Sex requires that someone initiate it, which presented a frequent challenge to the passive stance taken by hippies. Further, frequent drug use was viewed as reminiscent of the alcoholic culture of the older generation. It happened, it was tolerated, but it was not admired. So, the factor of remembering the '60s probably does not disqualify attendance, but another factor does so more accurately: If you don't remember which side you were on in the '60s, then you probably were not there.

The youth movement of that time was more than anything else a counterculture, a reaction against dominant values in the '60s. These immigrant values, such as a belief in self-sacrifice, were likely to be challenged in a period of affluence. Adding the hallucinogens, birth control, and the sense of betrayal by the Vietnam draft guaranteed a reactionary period. The form it took was guided by Frankfort School teachers, such as Herbert Marcuse, who themselves were reacting both against the fascism they fled in Germany and against the mass culture they faced in 1950s America.

The counterculture took every middle-class societal value and reversed it. It presents a dramatic opportunity to observe pendulemia in silly action. Making this comparison drives home the role of pendulemia in errors of judgment. Further, on a practical level, we all have clients still "pendulemically" stuck in some of the dichotomies below. To the extent that we are all inheritors of cultural wisdom, we therapists can locate ourselves also on these pendulums, sometimes to the detriment of our clients. (In the late 1970s, while the culture was still reeling from these issues, my colleagues and I taught these distinctions to counselor trainees as part of a program called the Change Agents Training Institute.)

The pendulum swings from:

- The dominant culture of the 1940s to the early 1960s
    - to the counterculture of the late 1960s and early 1970s
        - to an example of a third option, hopefully more balanced.
- Unpleasant feelings should all be avoided, versus
    - all feelings should be acted on, or
        - distinguish between past and present sources of feelings.
- Everything and everyone in neatly distinct categories, versus,
    - no conscious labels, everything just *is*, or,
        - preference for experiential and practical concepts.
- Structured gender and professional hierarchy at home and work, versus
    - no imposed structure, expecting automatic equality, or
        - create intentional, new structure when one wants to move beyond hierarchical patterns in business or personal relationships.
- Hide secrets about self as "dirty laundry," versus
    - no secrets allowed, openness worshiped as a virtue, or
        - celebrate differences among people in our lives, including the varying appropriate levels of intimacy and self-disclosure.
- Sex is dirty, save it for someone you love, versus
    - casual sex is obligatory as the gauge of emotional health, or
        - develop and enjoy one's own choices about when to say yes and when no.

- ○ Gender roles firmly established, versus
  - ⊙ no gender differences allowed, or
    - ☯ self-defined individuals, with group differences understood and appreciated without bias.
- ○ Self-denial and duty only to others, versus
  - ⊙ duty to self-fulfillment and viewing the self as a collection of needs, or
    - ☯ self-directed commitment (Daniel Yankelovich wrote about these three in his book *New Rules*).

Of course, values vary, and the reader may not prefer the third example to either of the first two in every case. Still, in each case, we can see that there is a movement from one extreme to another, with the third option thereby ruled out without consideration.

In the arena of ethics, we find a prominent recognition of pendulemia. Aristotle taught the logical mean as the solution to the emotional extremes in human traits. In his ethical system, the extremes are vices, and moral perfection is a logical practice of finding the middle. For example, courage becomes a mean between rashness and cowardice. Generosity is a mean between being profligate and being tightfisted. Productivity balances between obsession and sloth.

Perfectly beyond the pendulum

In the East, the Buddha taught his path of enlightenment as a "middle way" between the extremes of self-indulgence and asceticism. The prominent Jewish philosopher Maimonides crafted a distinct version of a golden mean consistent with Jewish ethics. There is a funny thing about the examples above: Notice how obvious they are when we notice them. It seems too commonsense. Yet just as happens generally with the stress–regress of state-rigidity, our recognition of pendulemia becomes slippery and elusive when we most need it, which is when we are in its throes. It then becomes part of the background of consciousness, like the pen in our pocket, the glasses on our face, and the watch on our wrist. It is so ubiquitous that it becomes unnoticed. It then is only part of the unnoticed ground, not the figure of attention. As therapists, we can bring it to the fore, first for ourselves.

Before helping others, we need to place these phenomena back into noticed figures of our own awareness, to help our clients to escape these traps. Most people experience the challenge of many dichotomous questions, which they will bring to us.

- ☯ Are people free or enslaved by involuntary forces?
- ☯ Are humans essentially good or evil?
- ☯ Is life good or bad?
- ☯ Is life meaningful or just a futile attempt at self-fulfillment?
- ☯ Is it more important to be true to myself or to belong with others?

Then, we have several therapy-related dichotomies. In light of a phenomenon-based Aikido approach, all the following are false distinctions:

- ☯ Are therapists to be emotionally neutral or emotionally caring about clients?
- ☯ Should our responses to clients' questions be passive or directive?
- ☯ Is the best therapeutic approach full of techniques or intuitively tuned in to the soul of each client?

Professionally, maybe more than are most other professionals, we are in the judgment business. Our clients wrestle with their own errors of judgment, whereas we must judge how to respond in order to take a useful role without taking over for them.

Because pendulemia presents a significant challenge to judgment, we must be able to fix it. Because it affects everyone, we can also begin to correct it in ourselves. Seen in this light, this entire text is an exercise in multiplying options and overcoming pendulemia about our careers. Pendulemia strategies are like the Tao metaphor of flowing water: They glide us into synchronized harmony with simple and balanced realities, removing us from mistaken cognitive dualities. For example, we can learn to neither passively accept nor aggressively fight the overwhelming barriers to our work as psychotherapists. Instead, from the beginning of this book, we have sought another approach: attaching ourselves to all the forces pressing private practice, riding their energy, then turning the thrust to our advantage in helping others as we become professionally free ourselves.

A Rapid Path to Multiplying Options

Most of us are already frequently applying a simple intervention for treating pendulemia in our clients. We use it every time we ask someone, "What else could you do?" You probably also already treat dichotomous thinking as a typical cause for errors of judgment, especially when good judgment is most stressfully crucial. What is more likely to be news is the following: This very insight about pendulemic thinking will provide a therapeutic space for our work beyond the false dichotomy of either running people's lives or being passive facilitators. For example, when I first introduce the activity of expanding the range of choices, I will often put it in the following words:

> As you probably know, I am not supposed to vote on what you do. In fact, in my opinion, no one but you gets a vote, although well-meaning friends usually can't resist. The way I see it, because you're the one who will pay the price for whatever decision you make, only you get a say in the decision you make.

> On the other hand, I find that, when people feel pressured about a choice, they start to think that they have only two options. Often the choice seems to be between "awful" and "terrible"! So my job is to multiply your options. When people choose from among a larger array of options, they're much more likely to do what they really want.

When speaking this way about discovering alternatives, we are simultaneously stepping out of the fallacious either–or of therapist neutrality/passivity versus therapist bias/command. The previous summary of our assisting in option testing celebrates our recognition that, without taking over people's lives, a therapist can expand their thinking to the degree that the best choice often becomes clear. By framing the option-testing process in terms of pendulemia, our client not only understands an important principle for lucid problem solving but also sees the point of skilled therapeutic coaching.

How to Use Pain: 'Increased Discomfort'

Another manner in which to address pendulemia is through Aikido strategies that involve harnessing pain itself. Paradoxically, the method for achieving this intentionally applies "increased discomfort," so that is the term we will use for it. The earliest therapist to speak about this in a related way was Viktor Frankl (for example, in *Man's Search for Meaning*), in his technique of "paradoxical intention," which became popular in the form of "paradoxical interventions."

All the strategies that are useful in freeing people from pendulemia must somehow help us to stop the whirl when we want to get off. "Increased discomfort" accomplishes this by fighting fire with fire—in other words, by increasing patterned thinking or distressed emotion in a way that short-circuits itself.

We often witness clients who are not literally stuck, in the sense that they do not stay in one place. Instead, they swing back and forth between two unpleasant states. Not surprisingly, cycling rigidity brings little advantage over static versions. People are completely as stuck and alternatives are just as unavailable, including the alternative of freely choosing the other side.

Fully in motion and fully stuck

As therapists often observe, people usually work on their rigid patterns with the same patterns, without knowing it. It is natural for people to feel depressed about their depressions, anxious about their anxieties, frustrated about their frustrations, and guilty about feeling guilty. This tendency maintains even when people swing between two disparate distresses. Guilt–blame is the most common of these. When people become fed up with blaming themselves, they swing to the other side, as Janice did in the earlier vignette. After acting out (or after horrifying oneself by imagining acting out), the person retreats into guilty self-recrimination. True to a pendulum, one side leads to another, but this occurs without the person being aware of it.

By way of illustration, imagine a person with an illness who is somehow taking the wrong medication. Suppose further that the medication is creating the exact symptoms that are plaguing the patient. As the symptoms get worse, the patient will naturally take more and more medication. A very common example of the "wrong medicine" is addiction, in which the habit now creates much more of the pain that it was supposed to relieve. The addicted person does not see this, because there was a time when the addictive behavior

More and more of the wrong medicine

helped, at least once. Accordingly, an old AA expression observes, "Alcohol gave me wings to fly, and then it took away the sky." The nature of dependency is that excessive use of some mood-altering behavior is creating significant trouble in a person's life, trouble that one seeks to soothe by resorting to more of that same behavior. Inside the illusion, the addict thinks that the cause of the pain is too little of the addictive behavior or not doing it exactly right, rather than seeing the feedback loop. Reliably, we can also notice pendulemia in addictive behavior, whether it is a binge drinker who periodically "goes on the wagon," or a love addict who periodically swears off romance.

In this addictive spiral, each distress feeling has led inexorably to more trouble. As a result, we may not think we could find any help from this distressed emotion itself. Fortunately, this is mistaken. This pendulemic process, like all of them, ensnares us through unawareness. Awareness makes all the difference when it comes to freedom, and when people learn to see the pendulum on which they are swinging, the picture changes. They get new options.

For those with active addiction, the first step in recovery includes overcoming pendulemia. Imagine if part of having a broken arm included not believing you had a broken arm. Then, once or twice a year, the arm seems to heal completely. You can do pushups, pull-ups, wave the arm around—no broken arm. If such was the case, no one would get it set! Addiction is like that. The third of the TAC screens for alcoholic issues ("**T**hree or more" to feel it, "**A**nnoyed" at some time by criticism of one's drinking, trying to "**C**ut down" at some time) is the attempt to "cut down." So when people admit that they are powerless over their "substance of choice" and their lives have become unmanageable, they are admitting the pendulum: all their attempts to swing into mock control are just preparations for the next swing into out-of-control behavior. Now, for the first time, they have a new option. They can avoid the first drink and thus get off the swing.

Not everyone has substance abuse problems; yet there are probably no true non-addicts. All of us may be addicted to varying degrees to our own rigid behavior patterns, fooled by pendulemia to stay on one side of the pendulum as if that protects us from the other side. This being the case, "increased discomfort" becomes a useful strategy for managing these non-substance addictions. It consists of sabotaging the "safe" side.

Sabotaging the safe side through "increased-discomfort"

This cognitive method aims to increase discomfort with the preferred side of a pendulum. Recall that Janice tried to remain as long as possible on the guilty side, as it seemed better than the embarrassingly angry side. Applying increased discomfort, we instead ruin the false security in taking refuge in the preferred side of the pendulum. Extending the pendulum metaphor, the longer one stays on any one side, the farther the pendulum swings to that extreme. As a result, the farther the figurative pendulum swings toward any side, the more force it will have on the downswing. This power, supplying momentum on the downswing, takes one far toward the other side, which is the very side the client hates the most. This is visually clear, fits the client's experience, and with explanation it dramatically changes the picture. After increasing discomfort with the illusory "safe" side, we can actually help people to fear their previous refuge. Their aversion to the "worse" side becomes associated with the other extreme.

What astonishing Aikido alchemy such awareness provides! Once a person clearly understands the pendulemic behavior pattern, the pain that had previously made the rigidity worse now begins to make it better. The following are several instances of self-talk

The art of the Aikido alchemist

that apply awareness of a behavior pattern to weaken it, by making the "safe side" a less comfortable place to hang out. Such awareness provides increased discomfort on one side, without then swinging one to the opposite pole (which is mentioned in parentheses). Keep in mind that these particular "increased discomfort" strategies work best for cognitively mediated patterns. For behaviorally driven conditioning—say, of anxiety—one can use a different approach, such as the one found in the next section.

- ☯ For guilt (versus blame): "People who are trapped by a guilt pattern are self-absorbed by it. It would make me feel too guilty to waste time on guilt, when that time could be used to help others." Alternatively, "The longer I wait until speaking up, the louder I'm going to be when I do."
- ☯ For anger (versus acquiescence): "Anger is going to stop bossing me around. I'm angry at anger for controlling me, and I'm not putting up with it."
- ☯ For anxiety (versus impulsiveness): "Taking planned steps moves me out of this danger, whereas fear makes me trip."
- ☯ For excessive suspicion or paranoid mistrust (versus misplaced trust): "Some people do not like me and are against me. I am too suspicious to let generalized suspicion keep me from clearly knowing who is and who isn't."

Although sabotaging the safe side is a powerful cognitive technique, the next version of "increased discomfort" is helpful even when cognitive clarity proves useless. This technique consists of *intentionally increasing an emotional experience in order to weaken it.* Even during a discussion of Aikido strategies, this sounds counterintuitive. Thus, it would be helpful to note the way that polar opposites work.

Trying to hurt so good

Most extremes have a limit in the healthy psyche. Except in deep pathology, extending a polarity sufficiently beyond a person's comfort level tends to reverse it. For some societal instances, see the sidebar.

In counseling sessions, taking a distorted form of thinking further than a person is willing to go can have dramatic therapeutic effects. It spontaneously and reliably stimulates a balancing mechanism. This suggests that our brains' wiring may automatically seek a kind of homeostasis or balance. You can experience this usefully in your sessions. If you find that someone has taken a strongly polarized position, extend that stand even further. If you take it far enough, the polarity will switch. A couple of treatment notes, however: Because of the importance of working in a peer style, I

Swinging the pendulum in sessions

Extending a Polarity Tends to Reverse It: an Example

Consider the rapid rejection of public anti-Semitism in the United States after World War II. It was widely considered acceptable to disdain Jews before that war. In fact, historians suggest that the American Nazi lobby had successfully inhibited Franklin Roosevelt in his acts to support England by casting the escalating conflict as a Jewish war over a Jewish problem. Even during the war, which only the bombing of Pearl Harbor had justified to the public, Roosevelt refused, despite requests, to bomb the tracks to the death camps. Some attribute this to his apprehension of this same impression, that such bombing would reveal the war as an attempt to aid Jews.

Yet after the war, the pictures came out, as well as the horrified first-person accounts of liberating soldiers, including future President

Continued on next page

suggest getting someone's permission before doing this, as I did in the example later in this section. On the other hand, as this example also shows, this Aikido technique can be literally lifesaving in the case of either too much or too little anger.

In the case of the danger of too much anger, Dr. Steve Simmer, a Massachusetts psychotherapist who has designed innovative anger workshops, suggests asking clients who are experiencing interpersonal conflicts for an assessment of the percentage of blame they would attribute to the person they are blaming. In doing so, he may encourage clients to assess blame excessively. For example, if the blaming person hesitates to give a number, the therapist might ask, according to this fictional illustration:

Is it all, 100 percent, her?

"Nothing's 100 percent anything. You can't say that."

Extending a Polarity Tends to Reverse It: an Example (cont.)

Eisenhower. The nation suddenly recoiled from anti-Semitism, being careful to label Judaism one of the country's three major religions, despite its relatively small numbers. Some would explain this in terms of Jewish contributions to the society, but those contributions did not originate after the Second World War.

Eventually, this public abhorrence of prejudice extended to race hatred. It did not yet extend to hatred of sexual minorities. In the 1990s mainstream people would still protest in public in opposition to human rights for gay people. What changed this? The most likely factor was public revulsion to the most shockingly violent attacks against gays. We saw the beginning of this pendulum reverse in public reaction to the slaying of Matthew Shepard in Laramie, Wyoming in 1998.

> *I understand. Well, what percentage would you give yourself, then?*
>
> "That's hard to say. How can you put numbers on that?"
>
> *Okay, well we're just being approximate, of course. How about 1 percent?*
>
> "It has to be bigger than that."

In this way, the angry person has begun to explore responsibility. By the way, as Simmer also points out, even a 5 percent sense of responsibility allows the therapist to suggest next, "Well, if you have a five percent role in the outcome, and you changed that five percent, could that have an effect on how things turn out? "

Too little anger can be dangerous too. A colleague referred Ryan to me because of this risk. He was feeling depressed to the point of having increasingly suicidal thoughts.

Too little anger can be deadly

His therapist became concerned about the risk and asked me whether I would treat him. In my first interview with Ryan, he showed a lot of self-insight. He had learned in his previous sessions, accurately, that he had unresolved anger at his ex-fiancée. She had suddenly jilted him, with no warning and little explanation, which in turn had touched off Ryan's depression. Cognitive insight was not availing him—he was still stuck. He sat across from me, with a clear and intelligent expression, despite his sluggish bodily movements. His eyes were perpetually moist, and his eyebrows drooped. After giving me a history of the relationship, the breakup, and his depression, he got to his dilemma.

> "I have been to two therapists, both of whom told me that I need to get my anger out. The last one, Dr. Cooper, went as far as saying that it might save my life, because I'm thinking of suicide. But I don't know how to feel what I don't feel."

Does anger about this seem to make sense to you?

"Oh yeah. I know I should be angry. I just can't get there."

If I could show a way to gain access to this anger, would you do it?

"I would do anything to feel better, if it worked, but nothing has."

I know how to get you to feel angry. People get angry with me all the time—just kidding. Actually, I am certain I can help you to feel the anger, but I need you to agree in advance to say whatever I suggest. I have to tell you that it involves repeating statements that you won't agree with.

"That doesn't seem too difficult."

Well, let's both agree up front that you may not agree with some of these statements, so that you don't have to tell me later, okay?

"Okay, fine."

At this point, I asked Ryan to repeat various sentences, directed toward his ex-fiancée, and to signal me with his hand if he started to notice any feelings of anger inside. I described angry sensations as heating of his skin, a burning sensation in his chest, and/or an itchy tension in his muscles. Statements that he was able to repeat several times without experiencing any of this included:

"I can accept what you did in leaving me."

"It's really okay with me that you left me."

"I don't mind at all that you threw away our relationship without a second thought."

"You are allowed to operate that way in your life, and I don't mind at all."

"You can do it all you want."

"You can do it to me again if you want to."

Not all people make it this far, but Ryan did. He reported not one sensation related to anger during any of this. I could see why his previous therapist considered his a difficult case. As for me, I was simply relying on the Aikido power of extending his pendulemia to rescue both of us. I took it to the next level.

Still nothing?

"Nothing."

Okay, now say 'Thank you for breaking up with me.'

"Thank her?"

Yes, exactly, 'Thank you so much for breaking up with me.'

"I can't say that!"

Of course, you don't believe it. That's the reason to say it.

"Thank you for breaking up with me." (*Gritting his teeth*)

Again.

"Thanks for breaking up with me." (*Eyes less moist*)

Good, again.

"Thanks for breaking up with me." (*Fingers gripping the chair*)

I want to thank you deeply for breaking up with me.

"I want to thank you deeply—Okay! Okay, I'm angry. What now?"

From this point, it was a simple matter of teaching him some modes of expression for his new-found and lifesaving feeling.

Some folks have too much anger; some have too little, as we have seen. Either extreme is heartbreaking, and sometimes even deadly. A depressed person may know he or she is angry, but low energy robs the readiness to find energizing anger. As we can see, *taking an emotional state beyond a person's tolerance tends to reverse it.* We even see this in the case of parody, in which exaggerating a serious emotional distress produces humor instead. Similarly, if a person can be convinced to attempt to increase all the sensations of anxiety, that anxiety tends to dissipate within minutes. Especially when we couple this kind of strategy with increased awareness, one can relieve a rigid emotional state without sending a person to the opposite extreme.

So far, using both the cognitive and experiential versions of increased discomfort, we have been working with one side of the pendulum to balance out experience. Next, we will work with both sides at once. We will be seeking a dynamic and rhythmic type of balance, which is not at all static. The Tao is never static. Recall the first example of the power of the Tao is that of water, the very power of which stems from its movement.

How to Ride Pain: 'Reciprocal Discomfort'

We all recognize that the middle road is best. Once again, we encounter a cliché that carries a valuable observation. So we hear: all things in moderation; seek the golden mean; find the middle ground; balance your priorities. All this sounds good, but brings a challenge. One reason we need to hear about balance so much is that achieving balance is elusive. A second challenge is to find a middle ground that is not mediocre. We will want a balance that is rhythmic in that it moves flexibly and combines the advantages from both sides. We will soon review a pendulemia intervention that produces such a rhythmic balance.

How to tune an untunable radio

We know from its reputation that the balanced place is supposed to feel good—if only one could find it. As a result, like beachcombers looking for a gold coin without metal detectors, people search back and forth between extremes waiting to feel good. It would be like trying to tune a radio in a spot with poor reception, where no station pops into clear transmission. When nothing happens, people become discouraged. The strategy of "reciprocal discomfort" presents a helpful alternative.

To understand it, we need to take a quick chemistry lesson. One need not recall the periodic table of the elements, just those charming little mechanical scales that measured the weights of material. I also find this metaphor very familiar to my clients. Whether it is from chemistry class, doctors' scales, or adolescent experience seeing drugs weighed, I do not know.

Recall how one knows when one has arrived at the correct weight for an item on one of those scales. One does not have to wait until the pointer stops moving. As soon as an observer notices that the pointer is moving past the zero point equally in both directions, the two sides are in balance. So, if it moves two marks past zero in one direction and then two marks past zero in the other direction, given enough time it would stop at zero.

The same principle works in search of Aristotle's ethical mean: Rather than search for perfect balance in some life area, we can find the point at which we seem to be out of balance equally in both directions. I usually call this gauge "reciprocal discomfort." To illustrate it, I will describe a childhood experience that gradually shaped my awareness of this balancing method.

As a child, I found school to be generally boring. I could not tell why many of my teachers were bothering to teach their subjects, as they did not seem very interested in the topics themselves. Because they were not at all intrigued, it escaped me why I should be. Sometimes, I overcame this through my own inquisitiveness; other times, I did not.

The aikido of a kid who did not like school

When I failed to generate intrinsic interest, I became interested instead in minimizing the attention that the class would require from me. I would gather all the information that we were mandated to know, having it available for later use. In some classes, but not always, I absorbed enough through temporary recollection to pass classroom quizzes. At the end of the semester, I would cram for exams. Making up a schedule, I divided all the class material into segments and proceeded to try learning it.

This is when I began to notice an odd experience. There were occasions when I prepared this study schedule too long in advance. The signal of this was a feeling of burning in my chest. I eventually realized that this was frustration, but I first supposed this meant that I just did not like studying. Then my further misadventures supplied more data. If I waited too long to study, I felt none of that burning in my chest. Instead, I felt a decided knot in my belly. I knew from other worrisome experiences that this was fear.

What amazed me was my discovery of a third situation. There seemed to be a certain amount of time before an exam during which I felt uncomfortable both ways. Although it was a milder and less uncomfortable version of each discomfort, there was no doubt that I felt some agitation in my chest and some gripping in my middle, both at the same time. Soon, I learned that, for some strange reason, if I began my study when I felt both discomforts reciprocally, I would have the exact time I needed to prepare for the exam.

The effect was so surprising, both to me and to a couple of my teachers, that I was once accused of cheating. This instructor, in whose class I had not spontaneously sponged up enough to pass the quizzes, could not believe my exam outcome. Even my explanation that I finally studied did not impress him. Only my offer to answer any questions he might have about course content, right on the spot, managed to save the day.

In the same way, "reciprocal discomfort" means feeling uncomfortable two ways. The strategy suggests that, for instance, if you feel only as if you are neglecting your work, then you probably are. On the other hand, if you feel only as if you are neglecting your personal life, then this is probably true as well. On the third hand, so to speak (as we are talking about moving beyond dichotomies), if you are feeling as if you are neglecting both elements of your life a little, and you feel uncomfortable approximately the same amount in both directions, then this is a good sign. You probably have found your own mean. This will not approximate everyone's balance, but just your own. Given enough time in that space, especially when you know where you are, it actually starts to feel good.

Twice uncomfortable is once balanced

This is a simple technique, which people can quickly learn and apply. Procrastination is a particularly relevant application, especially in the light of the many studies on the "inverted U-shaped curve" between stress and performance (Broadbent 1971; Duffy 1962; Kemeny 1979; Zajonc 1965). When we procrastinate, we typically swing between avoidance and panic. That, and not delay, is the mistake. Indeed, it is not a mistake to delay performing an important task until the stress climbs a bit. During overly low stress, we will likely perform errors of omission (Broadbent 1971), often called "careless mistakes."

The inverted u and You

On top of the performance curve is the sweet spot of moderate stress, commonly called "motivation." This is also practical information that our clients can apply immediately to forgive themselves for delaying tasks. After this forgiveness, we can help them find the right moment to perform the task, just as in the example of my childhood serendipity.

Another useful place to apply reciprocal discomfort is in helping certain people to become more "psychologically minded." One of the pendulums in common experience swings between the "dwellers" and the "avoiders." Many of us analyze our problems to the point of immobilization. Because of this pitfall, we have heard the expression that "analysis is paralysis." Of course, the person who coined that expression was probably of the opposite tendency. Those of us who avoid emotional content make a virtue out of the normal defense of denial. Even though denial is nothing to be ashamed of, neither is it a cause for a recognition award for impressive coping skills.

Dwelling with avoiders vs. avoiding dwellers

Of course, in true pendulemic style, dwellers and avoiders each point to the other to justify their own style. It is predictable to the point that it can be amusing. Suggest to an avoider that he or she get some counseling, and you are likely to hear, "So I can spend my life second-guessing everything I do? Right! There comes a time you just have to do what you have to do, not blame your childhood for every failing you have." On the other hand, we have all had clients who we actually wished would not work on the session content during the week. "Let *me* do more of the work," we tell them. Whereas the avoiders' slogan could be "Ignorance is bliss," problem dwellers insist, with Socrates, "The unexamined life is not worth living." Thereupon, they render the parameters of life coincident with their struggles, so life becomes, in fact, less worth living.

The balance, in this case, is lucid *awareness*. As therapists, we know that blaming one's past for one's future is immobilizing, not to mention irresponsible. We simultaneously know that those who do not learn from the mistakes of the past are likely to repeat them. The process of awareness glances at the past long enough to uncover the source of our rigid patterns. This allows us to attribute the old learning to its past usefulness, to see it as anachronistic, and to build a different future.

By applying reciprocal discomfort, we can gauge the usefulness of our awareness. Our periodic investigation of old and painful memories feels uncomfortable in a wistful way, but it is somewhat sweet because of the compassion for the children that we were. Meanwhile, our present-day adventures into new territory feel scary, but also a bit thrilling. If one maintains some of each type of discomfort, one most likely is neither a dweller nor an avoider. Instead, one has most likely harmonized awareness and action. In such balance, each of these types of discomfort brings its own therapeutic benefit. Let us take a closer look.

A handy way to gauge awareness

Benefits of the discomfort of awareness of the past. You have probably heard the expression, "You can't heal what you can't feel." That is because we cannot make real what we cannot feel. Re-experiencing pain about the past does not comprise the healing, but is a side effect of vividly remembering previous afflictions. Making the pain real returns access to the psychological premises lying unchallenged in traumatic moments, premises that otherwise define and confine future life. The process of making previous events real and allowing them to hurt again, in turn, elicits the pain of re-"member"-ing" the events by giving them arms and legs (members) again, temporarily. Our reward is that we begin to love ourselves as children, and to take our child-selves home with us. Through this contact, they get our wisdom and protection and we get their fresh awareness and vulnerability.

Benefits of the discomfort of action. On the other hand, operating from present-time freedom is a bit painful too. Although it is frightening, it is a refreshingly different kind of fear. The articulate philosopher Alan Watts once described this unfamiliar variety of freedom as "being out in the middle of the desert, with a fine automobile, a full tank of gas, but no road signs." We are in the freedom business, yet this freedom itself is scary.

As in the other cases of balance through reciprocal discomfort, our clients can learn to feel similar amounts of both kinds of pain, the pain from looking at the past and the pain from leaving the past behind. The best way to prepare our clients for this is by first informing them of the emotional cost of the journey. You are, after all, the travel guide to the affective scenery they are experiencing. As such, remember to preview coming attractions. *Reciprocal discomfort is the gauge, but freedom to achieve our life objectives is the destination.* Our clients tell us where they want to go, and our job is to know how to get there. Once you learn the type of transformation that you are coaching for someone, the balance between past awareness and future direction begins the path to getting there.

Incidentally, note how often we have seen that supplying therapeutic information can be highly helpful. *Because pendulemia insights are also Aikido strategies, they have the simple power of bringing us into synchronized harmony with straightforward realities, instead of our dichotomous conceptions of reality.* Fortunately, we work at a time when "psychoeducation" is now a valid modality. We can thank the cognitive–behavioral school of therapy for that. When I began working as a therapist, only the alcoholism counselors were teaching in sessions. They were AA-based and had no choice but to be effective in a hurry. They knew, often as

Talking therapists in talk therapy?

AA members themselves, that practical concepts were portable. Clients could take a pragmatic maxim out of a meeting or counseling session and into their lives. Today, neuropsychological researchers tell us that such learning, if reinforced, establishes new neural pathways in the brain, in this way effecting physical changes in the brain. In the same way, as we discover straightforward ways of articulating our Aikido insights, we must offer these to our clients also, because we also want our sessions to be effective in a hurry.

The best of these methods will be simple and intuitive. This simplicity of expression is not a form of disrespecting or patronizing our clients, of course. As is the case with AA slogans, the simplicity renders the insights readily available in periods of high stress, when we are all simple-minded.

Other Strategies for Progress with the Pendulum

In a lecture on the influence of childhood experience on adult choices, I once heard life described as being similar to trying to drive a car by only looking out the rear-view mirror. To apply another analogy, it can be hard for any of us to see outside the tunnel vision provided by the circumstances of youth, especially during the state of rigidity brought on by the stress–regress.

As I write this, I have just finished speaking to a woman who lost the affection of her entire family, which was totally her fault, as she would be the first to tell you. The surprise is that she is a highly principled and reliable person—a go-to, come-through kind of woman. In her work as a nurse practitioner, she demonstrates this daily, fully deserving her reputation for combining excellent skills with flexible attention to the individual

Reliving the past by repeating it

needs of each patient. Unraveling her contrasting personal choices has been an interesting challenge. She chose to have an open love affair, to see this as her destiny, to act blasé about its effect on her marriage and children, to then panic when all came to fruition.

This was when I met her, when she panicked. Her husband seemed beyond caring, whereas she was desperate to have another chance and was unable to forgive herself for making such a mess of her family. I thought I might understand her when I looked at her high standards for herself and when I learned that she had always disparaged cheating spouses. Of course, I figured, she could not allow her affair to be merely an affair; it had to be the love of her life.

This did not work for me, though. She should have exhibited guilt over her choices, in keeping with her scruples, if that is all there was to it. Then I learned more. Specifically, I learned three facts about her childhood: First, she was adopted; second, her adoptive father died when she was four years old, and her stepfather became her third "Dad." Finally, both her mother and stepfather drink plenty, and daily. This triple-whammy of abandonment could well explain her reenactment (called a repetition compulsion) in her marriage. She had to do everything she could to test whether it was possible to make her husband abandon her—and, of course, she succeeded.

These kinds of dramatic events confront us often in our attempts to free our clients from the past. Fortunately, a pendulemia-informed technique can provide the tools to come as close as possible to actually rewriting childhood history.

Rewriting past history

We can call this technique reconstructive regression. It consists of a modification of therapeutic work on the past that paradoxically keeps a present-time focus. If such a combination is possible, *it would overcome the pendulemia between past-oriented and present-focused therapy.*

There are several ways in which this reconstructive–regressive work keeps a balance between the present and the past.

- ☯ First, it does not use hypnotic regression as a method of retrieving memories. Rather, the regressive work glances at memories that the client mostly recalls in the present.
- ☯ Second, during the regression, the therapist asks the client to describe the details as if they are happening in the present, using the present tense. This deepens the experience and includes not only the interpersonal events, but also the physical details of the original setting.
- ☯ Third and most important, this method brings present-time skills into the past, in effect redeeming the client from the event. One method has the adult enter the past situation, in fantasy, to rescue the child. Another version has the child grow up from small to adult-sized right in the past fantasy, thereupon changing the outcome. Finally, the client can stay child-sized, but apply information now available from adult life to save the child.

This is not "wishful thinking." We are not altering persons and events originally confronting the child. In flooding the past with present-time skills, we are not altering those either. The adult really is more skilled and more powerful than the child was. We are only bringing the present and the past together. This strategy is so powerful that the process of describing it in a session is highly therapeutic in itself, as your client imagines this past–present reunion.

Another arena in need of pendulemic correction is the development of realistic, balanced self-esteem. In this case, the dichotomous extremes feature the awful choices of bashful self-effacement versus boastful arrogance. In contrast, self-appreciation is a balanced

Off the pendulum and into self-esteem

position in which people are encouraged to identify resources that were ever evident in their lives. The logic behind this is that any resource ever exhibited must be inside somewhere.

Far from becoming vain or boastful, this approach tempers self-appreciation with gratitude, even reverence. *Any thorough reflection on personal talents reveals that we merit very little simply by virtue of possessing them.* When we identify a knack for any endeavor, although it is up to us to develop it, we know that the original source is not in us. No matter how one defines the natural ground of being from which our lives spring, this is where any credit lies. As a result, we accurately call our talents "gifts." As a result, self-appreciation at its best does not vaunt one's own superiority over others. Rather, it acknowledges one's own life force and the ancient streams through which it flows.

Equipped with such an attitude, we can go exploring for personal treasure, as in the following analogy:

> Once upon a time, I climbed a mountain and found gold. Eventually, I forgot about it. Now, years later, I find that I have a need for that gold. I can remember once finding it, somewhere in that mountain. Even if I have forgotten where it was, I know that it is there. Maybe I could find it again.

In this way, our task in improving self-esteem and realistic confidence is a matter of searching for something that has been lost.

Actually you *can* be perfect!

You could say that what we need is a "missing qualities bureau." When I ask my clients to recall B-movies, they often recall the predictable questions: "What's his name? Where did you last see him? What did he look like?"

Correctly applied, self-esteem work not only improves a poor self-image, but can also help with the problem of perfectionism. This would be wonderful, because perfectionism is as harmful to self-esteem as is irresponsibility.

Defined in terms of pendulemia, perfectionism consists of the attempt to achieve an infinite extension into one side of a set of dual opposites. You could call this Platonic perfection, versus the Aristotelian sort (seeking the "golden mean"), which is the much healthier choice. In the psychologically destructive Platonic version, you choose the better of the two opposites and aim to be flawless in that extreme. Phrased this way, it hardly seems perfect at all.

If we look at the natural world around us—from the tree to the sunset to the mountain to the ocean—we can readily see that opposites work together in beautiful harmonies. Hardness and softness, brilliance and darkness, forcefulness and yielding all move together in exquisite patterns of a special kind of balance in which the opposites retain their full dynamism. We first looked at this expressed as "yin" and "yang" in the preface. People, on the other hand "are like a goat trying to be a goal," to paraphrase an ancient Taoist philosopher (Chuang Tzu). People often value one side of a set of opposites over another. Because one side helps our survival more than the other, this is a natural urge. Platonic perfectionism takes this tendency one step further. Believing that a particular side is not only useful, but also morally better, we seek a false and impossible perfection by aiming for unlimited scope on that one side. We will inevitably fail, since the world consists of the rhythmic movement of opposites described in the Tao, not the victory of positive over negative.

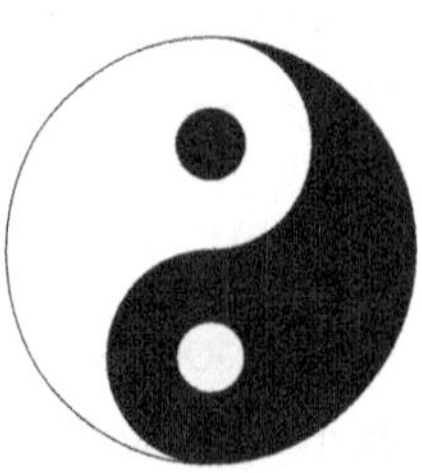

Recall the yin–yang symbol (also called the *Tai Chi* or "great Energy"). At the center of the dark principle is the birth of the light principle. At the greatest extension of either binary extension, the opposite is engendered. Rest leads to restlessness, which leads to activity, which leads to expended energy, which leads to rest. Although people must fail in any attempt to exemplify a perfect extreme, rigid beliefs persist regardless of facts. As a result, perfectionists agonize profoundly as they watch themselves failing.

To illustrate, let us outline the costs below. In each example, as one aims for and fails at achieving the first extreme of each set of opposites, one manages "perfectly" to lose the third, balanced alternative.

- ☯ Productivity, yes; pointless activity (play), no.
  Time for smelling roses loses.
- ☯ Youthful health, yes; aging and weakness, no.
  Wisdom loses.
- ☯ Powerful victory, yes; yielding acceptance, no.
  Aikido loses.
- ☯ Intelligent categorization, yes; emotional guesses, no.
  Intuition loses.
- ☯ Conforming to expectations, yes; mistakes and deviation, no.
  Creativity loses.
- ☯ Encyclopedic competence, yes; lack of knowledge, no.
  Learning loses.

As clients learn this perspective, *perfectionism becomes an imperfect endeavor.* As perfectionists, therefore, they naturally begin to reject it. Isn't Aikido grand? Now they are in position to learn a new way to model self-esteem, a process that you have already positioned as an act of gratitude rather than vanity.

However, we still have to contend with one important contradiction in our attempts to avoid the Platonically imperfect version of perfectionism. It begins as we go looking for our innate gifts. As soon as we start to measure our abilities versus other people's, we enter a dual,

Jumping off the scale and onto the snowflake

Platonic universe: measuring up or not measuring up. How can we identify our positive qualities without such perfectionist pressure? If the positive qualities that we each reveal are not best calibrated on a dial of Platonic perfection, how are we to assess them?

Calibrated self-assessment produces either vanity or shame; discovering our unique "configurations" instead produces gratitude for our gifts. Who has the most perfect nose in the world? Is it possible to judge this? If it were, this could be an achievement of sorts for one person. Meanwhile, although only one person in the world could possibly (but inconceivably) be rated as the one with the most perfectly formed single facial feature, each of us has a unique face. Similarly, only one person in the world could ever achieve a rank as the ultimate in any specific positive trait. If we agreed on the criterion and if we held a worldwide contest, perhaps we could crown one person as embodying a type of ability most fully. Perhaps the Olympics most successfully achieve this—but even there, only ephemerally.

As a result, other than for premier athletes in the temporary and circumscribed arenas of their performance, such calibrations do not help us or anyone else we know. On the other hand, we are all unique in our particular combination of abilities. There are not only many varieties of any gift we may possess, but also an endless array of talents. We are like snowflakes. Thus, each of us is essentially unparalleled in our constellation of abilities, all of which coalesce into the unique opportunity of each person's life.. Understanding this, we can teach it to our clients. From this balanced position, we can nurture the growth of a self-esteem that insulates our clients from anxiety and depression, while encouraging their responsibility to develop their talents and share them with the world.

Notice the Aikido element of this kind of self-appreciation, flowing with each of our innate and unique inheritance from the universe, with the result that we are no longer judging ourselves on some imagined

Surfing one's way to self-esteem

scale of comparison of ourselves with others. This is good news, as we can usually find many people superior to each of us on any one dimension we might question. Instead, we can learn to draw the contours of our individual highs and lows, generating a cocktail of talents, all creating a unique flavor and comprising a potent potion with which to contribute to life.

In practice, besides explaining the significant difference between calibration and configuration, we can provide homework exercises to develop this awareness. One approach is to literally *draw the contour of each person's abilities on a chart.* To begin, list qualities along the left margin. They can be open-ended adjectives, which allow people to decide how they envision and fit each dimension. Words such as "sparkling," "diverse," and "quick" can fit among more common typically sought qualities, such as "intelligent," "witty," and "warm." To assist a configuration consciousness, rather than the chart using ratings of low to high, the small change to "lower" and "higher" shifts the focus of the assessment so that each trait is low or high relative to the others one possesses, rather than being a comparison with those of other people. Here is the list that my former colleague, Tom Sargent, developed:

> Intelligent, diverse, deep, accurate, warm, versatile, enthusiastic, responsive, alive, easy, solid, committed, determined, precise, generous, sparkling, creative, curious, coordinated, strong, flexible, thorough, confident, quick.

Another strategy, useful with both older children and adults, is a *self-esteem journal.* We ask people to identify one event daily that they either enjoyed or did well. Second, they write a feeling state associated with the event—a term such as *excited, confident, peaceful,* or *close.* One of those two—the event or the feeling associated with it—will next reveal a personal talent. If the event is an example of high performance, the question becomes "What would you say of someone else who did that as well?" If the event is, instead, about not performance but enjoyment, then the positive quality comes from seeing the kind of person who would feel that way. So, if I wrote the music, I can appreciate how I did it. If I only listened to it, I can appreciate my capacity to enjoy it in the way I did.

Perhaps, when we first began considering ways to find a rhythmic balance between opposites, you immediately thought of couples. If individuals can swing back and forth in cycling pendulemia or become stuck in frozen pendulemia, then couples can embody two battling extremes at once. There is an expression that couples split up for the same reasons that they originally got together, so opposites originally attract and then repel. As a result, to the extent that we work with couples, we already engage in a search for a complementary harmony to help them. Sometimes this effort is sufficient; sometimes it is not. In fact, as we will see, we may not be able to resolve all struggling marriages by focusing on differences alone.

Pendulemia à deux

In the 1990s, an interplanetary metaphor descended on us and soared heavenward in the media. John Gray did a splendid job of simplifying some complex communication issues between the genders. Some of his best observations followed the excellent gender comparisons made by Deborah Tannen, a psycholinguistics professor at Georgetown University. Her books, *You Just Don't Understand* and the workplace version, *Talking Nine to Five,* lay out the gender differences that plague heterosexual couples.

These are useful clarifications. *Spouses can more easily rebuild trust once they take these gender-based misunderstandings less personally.* Identifying what might be called "common couple communication conundrums" relieves the need to blame one's spouse or the relationship. Yet there is more to the picture than interplanetary warfare.

As we just noted, differences appear both to attract couples together and repel them. So, what happens? A fascinating hypothesis is that *couples do not truly conflict because of their differences, but because of their similarities.* This, of course, bears some explanation.

Romantic attraction is based on more than differences. Initially, people get together because of certain attractive personality differences and other important similarities on dimensions such as values. Differences in personalities plus similarities in priorities could seem a magic formula for compatibility. Yet no two people are different in *all* personality dimensions. There is bound to be some overlap, in which any two people are going to be similar. Both may be exceptionally courteous, or particularly assertive, or admirably self-reliant. These are positive qualities.

The mosaic principle of common ground

Still, an asset or liability is often a matter of where you see it. Each mutual similarity between romantic partners also leaves some area in which there is no one to fill in. For two people to make a life together, at least one party must be able to:

- Make decisions.
- Reach out for affection.
- Look for compromise.
- Plan joint activities.
- Lighten the atmosphere.
- Show appreciation.

- Initiate communication.
- Say no to impulsive choices.
- Bring up problems.
- Place conflicts on a concrete level for solution.

This may look like a long list, but most of this happens without thought for many couples. Various types of personality are more or less likely to do each of these things, but usually someone can cover most of these needs. On the other hand, there will inevitably be areas of common ground to both personalities. This results in an unfilled position in the couple, so to speak. Picture two mosaics of the same picture, each of which has colored pieces covering most of the surface, yet with some missing. Now overlay one mosaic on top of the other. Some of the mosaic shapes will be filled twice, some only once, and, inevitably, one or two will still be left blank.

As a result of this, a very courteous couple may both be too polite to bring up problems; the assertive couple may not include a member who looks for compromise; the self-reliant couple may not have anyone to whom to reach out for affection. What happens instead? It is difficult for people to fight over similarities, so no one will complain at first. What can one say? "I hate that you are like me!" does not work for an argument. Instead, the spouses will become more irritable with each other, until someone voices displeasure. Whether this is a hot war or a cold war, despite the cause, the content of the argument will be about differences, not similarities.

Thus, we now have two models of couple conflict. The "opposites attract and repel" hypothesis pits one polarity against the other and seeks adjustments and compromises. The "common ground" hypothesis suggests that couples will feel an urge for conflict because of tension stemming from similarities, which they will voice instead as being over differences. Identification of this has remarkable power for couples. It places them back in harmony, in acceptance of their own natures; it also places them in synchronized momentum with the similarities in their spouses. As they ride this Tao wave, you have linked their commonalities and joined them in the next task of filling in the gaps together. As they both affirm the area of similarity, they begin to forgive the other for having the same limitation, and they recognize that both had better stretch toward filling this hole.

This model is speculative; I have nothing but anecdotal data for it. Rather, I discovered it by replaying moments of especially powerful breakthroughs with couples who had previously been stuck and not progressing in therapy. My observations of these moments then solidified into a conscious strategy with greater efficacy. Perhaps you will find it similarly useful. Further, it is a noteworthy example of a Tao technique for overcoming pendulemic polarities by finding middle ground, this time common ground already existing between members of a couple.

A Stance that Corrects the Dangers of Competence

Having a powerful armamentarium of strategies is a gift, as long as we do not excessively focus on finding a strategy during sessions instead of really seeing the person in front of us. The time to think about a technique is when we do not need to use it. Our goal, instead, is a flexible application of technique.

Imagine that you have programmed many of these and other strategies into your skill set, well in advance of needing them. Now that you are prepared in this manner, you enter the therapy room.

What is your metaphor about what happens next? Are we to become like a complex, elaborate computer, rapidly testing various options until we chance on the right combination? This might occasionally be practicable but it has several concomitant problems. First,

Beyond technique: two-feet therapy

we will lose our personal presence and come across as technicians. Most clients cannot build a working alliance with a machine. This is one of the reasons that you still have not been replaced by a computer program. Second, we can do much better.

Picture a different metaphor. Suppose that you have two feet—so far, so good. Now, imagine that you have one foot stepping fully into your client's life, without reserve. With this foot, matched Aikido-like to the position of your client, you identify openheartedly with the experiences brought to you. In the same way that you "suspend disbelief" to get the most out of a dramatic presentation, you make the experience of your client fully real for you. This is really not difficult. If we are even capable of identifying with a fictional character on the screen, how much more can we do so with the nonfictional person who is speaking deep truths about his or her life?

The innate experience that you have when you do this could be called "method therapy" if we make an analogy from "method acting." In method acting, the actors write notes along the margin of the script about related experiences from their own lives. As they say lines that do not usually come from their own lives, they are reliving parallel emotions from comparable moments that do come from their own experiences. The result of this effort is not that you will know exactly how your client feels, and you would never claim to do so. *You are just feeling your version of what you felt, at the times during which you went through the most similar events you can find.* Your emotional state is not identical with that of your clients, but becomes noticeably and powerfully congruent.

This allows the person in the client-role to become receptive to your suggestions. The price of admission into such receptivity is your willingness to feel your version of the other person's pain. It has been said that if you breathe exactly in rhythm with someone else, you can change the pace of the other person's breathing by altering yours.

Similarly, if you feel "in pace" with someone, that person will grant you access to changing those feelings.

Now, what about the other foot? If you go all the way over, with both feet, into people's experience, they will appreciate you, but you will not help them. In such a case, you have perhaps become a close friend, but not a therapist. You will be resonant, possibly popular, but relatively useless. Therefore, *it is important to keep one foot back in the rest of your own life, in the parts where you have lots of useful information, such as how to resolve problems.*

If we extend the movie analogy of suspending disbelief, this is how you watch gory scenes, assuming you can bear them. Researchers have found that people who can cope with graphic violence in film usually do so by removing themselves as much as necessary from the plot. They begin to analyze the special effects, for example, wondering how the film producer created the scene. In other words, they distance themselves just enough, accessing information from outside the movie experience. Keeping a foot in and a foot out of the experience of the movie, we manage to watch the film without the trauma of believing that we have just actually seen death or mutilation in front of us.

In this way, we may already have the skills to keep one foot in and one foot out of our clients' lives. By doing this, we are wonderfully overcoming our own pendulemia as therapists, transcending the extremes of both cold analysis and helpless overidentification. Instead, we are seeking a rhythm in which we fully experience our own versions of their struggles, while our cache of useful strategies also remains available to us—and, more important, to them.

Become a spontaneous warrior of transformation

Another useful analogy for this balance comes to us through the writings of D. T. Suzuki (in his chapter "Zen and Swordsmanship" in *Zen and Japanese Culture*). He describes the relationship between Zen meditative practice and sword fighting. Even though most of us hope never to have to master the use of a long sword, any approach that works well in as stressful an encounter as combat is naturally impressive to us. Zen practice, which refers to a focused type of awareness, became popular among the samurai warriors because it helped them survive. The way that Suzuki describes the Zen approach to sword fighting sounds much like our description of powerful therapy.

As we noted in a sidebar in Chapter 2, Zen is a marriage of the meditative school of Buddhism (dyana) with Chinese Taoist philosophy. This system is pronounced Ch'an in China and Zen in Japan. The Zen-trained warrior approaches combat with flexibility, full attention, and freedom from distractions. Even thoughts of the outcome of the event cannot distract the Zen swordsman from the present. Yet success does not result from the quality of such attention alone. As Suzuki explains, a Zen master who had not thoroughly studied sword technique would be "instantly defeated." This is our objective also. We are becoming fully accomplished in strategies, while being present and attentive during sessions. To return to the our first image of the same achievement, imagine that you are balanced between having one foot matching your client's life and one foot inside your own training. This is the best way I know to become a warrior of transformation.

4

The Tao of Running Your Psychotherapy Practice

Bringing It All Back Home

We are now in reach of the rest of our original goal—harnessing the factors hindering your practice and using them to your advantage. In service to this goal, we have just explored the alchemy of transforming the barriers to change, such as pendulemia, to actually assist in accomplishing transformation. Earlier, in the introduction, we mentioned that managed care can actually invigorate practice by allowing us to pour our hearts into our missions as therapists, while the corporations keep our weekly schedules (caseloads) in check. We will now turn to the nuts and bolts, such as how to set up a time-efficient long-term therapy practice, strategies for keeping one's independence while dealing with managed care, and methods to incorporate the strategies in this book both into one's theoretical paradigm and into one's sessions.

This is a somewhat dangerous part of the presentation. One danger is endemic to the search for specific methods itself; the other is endemic to business itself.

Any practice strategy that is not in harmony with your particular nature or with the general principles of helping people to change destroys the Aikido focus that we have been building. For example, when we discuss diversification, the point is not to scramble around for a way to stay in practice. On the contrary, *the point is to express what you love, and have the successful practice be a side effect.*

Second, in terms of the business concerns, let me be blunt: Don't try to make money! Obviously you are going to notice the condition of your business bank account, but do not stay there. Like a person in meditation who treats alien thoughts as clouds passing in a bright blue sky, return your focus to taking your best care of people and letting them notice that on their own. Otherwise, your extrinsic motivation will overtake your intrinsic motivation, and you will forget why you got into this field at all.

Because of the business factors we are about to discuss, we must first reemphasize this point: The strategies that follow are not instructions on how to make a living. You don't have to try to have a good practice; by practicing the Tao of psychotherapy, your results will grow your practice without your concerning yourself about it. In contrast, being financially

Despite the rationale that I am presenting, my suggestion not to try to produce income may seem like the optimistic speculations of a social scientist, so I am bringing in supportive evidence from an expert in the field of finance and marketing, Michael Phillips. As an executive at Bank of America, he cofounded its marketing research department and founded their Bank PR and Marketing Research Foundation. In this role, he became instrumental in developing MasterCard. He has written about a dozen business books, one of them called The Seven Laws of Money. The first of these laws, which he calls both the most important and most difficult of the seven, is: "Money will come when you are doing the right thing…Worry about your ability to do it and competence to do it, but certainly do not worry about the money."

focused will break the rhythm. How do you achieve this focus on service rather than compensation? If you cannot care deeply enough about your clients, you need to get additional treatment yourself to learn what has walled up your heart. Otherwise, just affectionately enjoy and deeply admire your clients—they are brave and wonderful people, taking responsibility for their lives, and willing to take a chance on change. After that, you can leave yourself out of the picture, because they will take care of you. Your clients will know authenticity when they see it; otherwise they would not be your kind of clients.

The techniques discussed in the following sections are just the details of how this preferable focus on contribution plays out.

Why Successful Practice Can Be a Breeze

Before we move into the details of your practice options, I will offer some of the details of my personal practice story. You may find this encouraging as you set your own direction. On the other hand, my bias toward a very independent practice is evident, and I recognize that you may or may not resonate with it.

In my view, the insurance industry tends to be a cynical world that washes away the evidence that psychotherapy is helpful, in favor of a rationalization that what is good for short-term profits is good for patients. Fortunately, this corporate cynicism may not include all the staff that you deal with on the phone. As we will see, the caseworkers often feel as trapped as you are and may even help you if you give them a way. However, you do not meet their chiefs, and these industry leaders prefer it just that way. They enter your practice not through the front door, but through the deception of "managing care." Still, I recall clearly that day that I saw this bleak assassin first enter my office.

At the time, I was the most afraid that I ever was about the encroaching power of HMOs. Every time I went to a psychologists'

The Accidental Taoist

meeting or bumped into a colleague, all I heard was the shrill chords of doom. The drums were beating, and I learned that private practice was already under assault. A professional plague had come upon us and had infected our appointment books and billing statements. It was too late to run, and there was nowhere to hide. There would be no one to save us, no cavalry to fight for us. Join or die fast as a private-practice therapist. "Join and die slowly," I thought. Still, I had better join a little.

Moreover, I had an "in." One of my referral chains were people involved in preparing CIGNA, one of the main insurers in the Hartford area, to "go HMO." That was good, as I had already missed the boat a bit. When I had finally checked into the first large HMO a couple of years earlier (Consititution Health Network, it was called), it was closed to new providers. I actually joined a small one, a Connecticut company called Liberty Health Plan, which went out of business, and I was rejected by a third, ConnectiCare, for having a nonhospital internship.

So, my connection with CIGNA seemed fortunate. It was, but in the opposite direction I had imagined. They said no also, because they preferred group practices. As a result, I admitted to myself that I did not like what was going on in the market, that my feeble attempts were fear-driven and uncommitted, and that I was not willing to do what others were doing. For example, I would not be joining a group practice in order to enter CIGNA HealthPlan. From then on, I decided to do what worked better for me. I wanted to see if I could sail through.

Awakening on a sailboat

I would let the forces around me determine my direction, but not by fighting them and not through submitting, but by letting the barriers shape my efforts. My choice was to apply the pressures around me, to sculpt a well-chiseled practice that would not dissolve but instead reveal its polished form under their onslaught. If water can make stones smooth, then managed care could shine my practice.

By the time that enrollments became more liberal, I was ready. I refused Blue Cross and all the other offers that came later. Meanwhile, I paid full attention to the fear tactics they used, such as the letter from Blue Cross letting me know that they would pay me directly only if I signed up. In effect, they were insulting my clients, implying it would cost me less to join them than for me to try to collect the reimbursement checks owed to me. I also noted carefully which people, of those referred to me, became scared off by my fee when compared with a fifteen-dollar co-pay without any deductible, versus those who had the opposite response.

Speaking of opposite responses, full attention to the fearful evidence had an opposite effect of pushing me toward greater resolve. In fact, it made me alert and charged me with a mandate to miss none of this experience. Instead, I focused on all of it: the fears, the joys of transformational moments in my office, the phone calls to my voicemail from prospective clients. Ultimately, I used all these forces to reveal the Tao of a post-HMO practice. The stumbling blocks became veritable stepping-stones and, through Aikido, the opposition became inspiration. It worked, and it worked better every year. In truth, I overflow every day with gratitude for the kind of practice these experiences blew into my life. This is how I decided to provide sailing lessons for other psychotherapists.

How Phenomenal Tao Focus Brings Us the Best of Every Therapy Style

Let us begin to explore the details of Aikido-inspired practice strategies with a meta-view of our theories. Theoreticians often have a tough time agreeing on how the mind works and how to help it work better. Here is why: *The mind does not work just one way.* There is an essentially dual nature to human experience. In some ways we are freer than the angels and in other ways we are more constrained than machines. On one hand we can sometimes go against every influence on us—whether that of history or genetics or social pressure—and innovate miracles. On the other hand, we lack the "erase" button that even a calculator has, so we often make the same mistake repeatedly, even when it counts—especially when it counts.

Duality such as this provides contradictory data and confuses psychologists. As a result, one group, the psychodynamic group, insists that we are enslaved by our instincts. This group is the smallest. Meanwhile, a large group, the cognitive–behavioral faction, sees us as similar to computers, just very complex if slow models, and programmed as such. A third group, the humanists, believes that we are potentially spiritual and ultimately free. The humanists have the most fun, but they are often the least useful in making change happen, because they do not deal too much with the automatic side of the human experience. Unfortunately, the psychodynamic group sees life itself as a disease, a profound war between selfish urges and civilized expectations. The cognitive–behavioral group is predominant in the literature, as it is the easiest to research, but, among other problems, you must see yourself as a computer to accept their help. These are very broad brushstrokes, with significant developments in each system, but the tendency to see the mind through a single lens persists.

The Tao, once again, opens up new options. In harmony with the polarities of yin and yang, both science and experience reveal that the life of the world is a life of duality. Perhaps the brain is dual also. We know that the neurons are. The operational balance of the brain is

The Tao of your brain

based on the balance of electrical and chemical elements in the firing of neurons. The brain also expresses the duality of a balance between the left brain and the right brain, and the balance between neuronal receptor sites and the hormones that stimulate them. For example, the brain's role in cocaine addiction involves reducing the responsiveness of the neural keyholes (seeking homeostasis) that the cocaine is trying to overstimulate. As another instance, when glucocorticoids (stress-related hormones released by the adrenal cortex) stimulate the hippocampus (the brain's "filing clerk"), the latter has a bimodal response. The first response to the rise in these hormones is to tell the brain, "Make good memories!" If the hormone level is too high, however, the instructions change to "Make fuzzy memories!"

Finally, the brain is also bimodal in terms of the stress–regress that we noted above. Brain imaging technology enables us to see it in action (LeDoux 1998). The brain, once again, works in balance of two modes, which result from two roads of response. During moderate stimulation (increased yang), the brain awakens to fully expanded awareness. In this state, yin responses, such as creative exploration, are in balance with yang responses of decision making and action. As the stress becomes too high for comfort, however, the brain moves into the rapid-response mode. The brain's response pathway becomes literally more compact (yang), so the thalamus (the "dispatcher") sets off the alarm center in the amygdala for what LeDoux calls "a quick and dirty response."

In this manner, the brain does not work one single way. It reveals the functional fluidity of the Tao. The nature of mental functioning during yin states of overly low stress will tend toward creative reverie, but will be unproductive. Balanced states of moderate stress will reveal the full capacity of the brain, but the yang pressure of emergency will elicit rapid, uncreative (automatic and regressive) responses.

This underscores the typical error of theoreticians in trying to ascertain how the brain works. If you are walking around with a hammer, everything starts to look like a nail. What can we do when the phenomena of life do not fit within the narrow framework of our concepts? I suggest that we can assemble all the significant concepts, each being useful in its way, on the flexible structure of our phenomenal awareness. If we can succeed, we would be achieving true theoretical integration.

Psychotherapy integration is a deservedly beloved goal for therapists. So many strengths stem from each of the major models. Who would want to toss them out because they do not fit one's own model? Although practical integration gets a lot of attention, theoretical integration has been elusive. This occurs because each of the theories rules out one or more of the others. If one begins with a Tao-like phenomenal focus, rather than working back from a theoretical stance, the picture changes remarkably.

Finally: true theoretical integration

The phenomenon of the stress–regress shows us a brain in which each theory is correct when it is correct, which is when the bimodal condition of the brain works that way. In other words, there are a way and a time in which psychodynamic theory is correct and useful: During stress, the regression is indeed back to past patterns, with childhood learning being the most dominant in more profound stress. The cognitive approach is helpful when these old, anachronistic patterns include distorted thinking, as they usually do. The behavioral approach steps in to assist us when these old patterns are so wired in that cognitive insight is insufficient to break them. Our humanistic visions provide the purpose for the freedom we seek and help make us more resilient to the effects of stress. They are all correct and helpful, and need not be mutually exclusive. *In the phenomenal light of the bimodal stress–regress, relatively minor modifications (such as making regression normal and an often short-term state of mind) allow us to incorporate fully the power of each contribution seamlessly in the same session.*

On the other hand, let us see what happens in the current monolithic approach to theory. Castonguay et al (2004) performed research on improving cognitive–behavioral therapy (CBT) results when there is a rupture in the therapeutic alliance. How did they improve results? They deleted the CBT manual section on strategies to handle such ruptures in the alliance. The CBT approach (which is cognitively stuck in its own theory) is to analyze further the causal relationship between a client's thoughts and his or her feelings about the therapy experience. If the client were enjoying this, however, the alliance would not be in trouble to begin with. Instead, Castonguay and colleagues applied such commonsense responses as empathy (listening and acknowledging what a person is feeling), inquiry (asking for elaboration), and disarming (finding any truth in another's perspective), which they took from the humanistic camp.

Integrating versus disintegrating therapy

Thus, there are practical reasons to find a way to integrate into your work everything that works. As we can see, it is not that any of these groups is wrong. The problem is exactly the opposite: They are all correct, in fact. This possibility does not occur to us most of the time—or if it does, it seems patently impossible So, we think we must choose one incomplete model or another. In fact, these models fit together surprisingly well, and we now see how. They are phenomenally linked in the yin and yang of our brains and linked, as though through a theoretical hub, by the bimodal phenomenon of state-rigidity. Keep in mind that when they are each correct, you can access the benefits of each without changing your mindset.

The Tao Guides Our Practice Strategies as It Guides Our Therapy Strategies

During our discussion of pendulemia, we noted the inverted U-shaped curve between stress and performance. This inverted U phenomenon has also been termed the Yerkes-Dodson law, and it shows that performance is best under moderately high stress. As we move into practice strategies, this effect on performance can help us understand the hidden power behind an Aikido-synchronized practice. In other words, we can operate such that our work offers more than it would have without the pressures on us. Even though the managed care-dominated practice environment supplies overly high stress without the Aikido approach, with the quiet assurance of the Tao response we can bring the heat down to the warming range. The win–win of this is that:

- ☯ The pressure keeps us sharp and fit, working with more intensity and satisfaction than we would achieve if times were fat and easy.
- ☯ We avoid the boring routine of HMO participation, which offers us a substandard arrangement but securely full schedules. This would comprise overly low stress on the Yerkes-Dodson curve.
- ☯ Stress is managed through confidence. You will see that you have created a practice that offers a much better therapeutic opportunity, so enough people will choose to see you rather than someone on their provider list.

On my web site, *www-dr-rick.com,* I inform prospective clients about this directly. I advise them as follows:

Pick a psychologist who does not take your insurance

Why should you do that? Because it can *save you money* and get you *better results* in the long run.

In psychological terms, a statement like that is what's called counter-intuitive. In other words, you might assume that the opposite is true. Or, putting it differently, I had better explain this or you'll think I'm making no sense!

Paradoxically, it makes a lot of sense. The reason is simple. When your out-of-pocket share of the bill is greater, it means I have to prove myself more quickly and provide recognizable results in addressing your important issues. That really sharpens my motivation and incentive, since I have to merit being an out-of-plan psychologist.

On the other hand, a psychologist who is in-plan is less pressed for results. This can lead to simply "running out the clock" and using up the client's benefit allotment. That could stretch out the time before you receive a treatment benefit (if it comes) and that can end up costing you more in co-pays. It also takes up a lot more of your valuable time.

This treatment paradox is exactly why I decided long ago not to become a member of the insurance plans. I realized that, by being an independent but licensed practitioner, I could be beholden strictly to my clients and address their needs most expeditiously. I would bill insurance companies out-of-plan, but I wouldn't have to kowtow to an insurance company limiting your treatment. Plan-member practitioners do, or they face being kicked out of the plan. I just couldn't see how I could coach people in bravely confronting crucial issues in their lives if I had to play it safe with the insurance companies to save my practice.

Continued on next page...

...Continued from previous page

My gamble in staying independent paid off, and my practice remains full. In fact, taking my stand has only pushed me to higher standards. People choose my services because of the unusual benefit of my practice style.

I often hear from new clients that I get much more done in every session than they had expected or even imagined before they met me. People frequently discover that they can see me a lot less than they thought would be necessary. If you clearly can benefit from more sessions than your insurance company wants to dictate, I can fight for those sessions without fear of being tossed out of the plan. I'll be working on your side, for your issues, all the way.

Here's the bottom line for you:

Since overcoming the pain of being personally stuck and achieving the joy of life-progress are the most important factors, choosing out-of-plan becomes a win-win situation for the people who see me. You can truly *save money and get better results* in the long run. Candidly, the most motivated and intelligent people of those who find me seem to come to the same conclusion that I have: "You have to be pretty good to be able to be busy and not 'take' insurance." It is thrilling for me to be able to work with these kinds of people.

You may be one of them.

In this way, I take the potential barrier of maintaining independence from participating provider lists and present it, Aikido fashion, as the therapeutic benefit that I deeply believe it is. Part of how this works is that *the many advantages of an Aikido-informed practice make it cost-effective for the people we see.* The excellence we can develop makes us surprisingly affordable without the impoverishment of insurance company control. For example, it allows us to operate within the treatment modality discussed in the next section.

How to Be Affordable without Becoming Poor

The time-efficient long-term (TELT) treatment modality is a central option for providing such value. *When you offer this option, many more clients can afford you, even if they see you only once a month.* It is not optimal for anyone in the sense that more frequent contact is, of course, beneficial. Further, it is not possible initially if someone is in crisis. However, I present it as an option to my clients after we move out of crisis, if more frequent contact is not feasible. Your Aikido-influenced demeanor produces a powerful alliance, which allows a lot to occur in each session. Meanwhile, your high-impact strategies give your clients something to take home with them. They can have plenty to do for a month, if they are willing. They can call or e-mail you for very brief conversations if they have any questions, and they return in four weeks for the next step in their growth.

At first, this TELT practice does not look like much. One client a month does not yet inspire one's independent urges. One client cannot provide security any more than one penny can provide wealth. Yet if you double that penny every day, you will have more than $10 million in one month! Building an independent practice is not literally a double-your-penny endeavor, but it does reveal some of the same geometric properties because of the referral factor. This frees you to work at your current job, and because this does not require extra time to build your practice, you need not be concerned over the pace. Be assured that there is no question that it can be done. Using these exact methods, I have continued to regenerate a fully independent practice for decades, regardless of economic cycles. Without participation in any managed care panels and without discounted fees, I have enjoyed a full practice of thirty-four sessions each week since I opened my practice in 1986.

How does one design such a business? Or, as we ask our clients, if we were going to do it, how would it look?

To Build a Successful Practice, Base It on Contribution

First, the practice would look service-oriented. If you are going to deinstitutionalize your practice, if you are going to build it free from participating-provider referrals, you must build it based on an attitude of overflowing contribution. This means that you are going to provide a higher standard of service for your clients; this assistance includes more than just the quality of your counseling.

For example, it is preferable that you offer *free billing services* for your clients. You also may want to suggest, not just allow, *phone calls between sessions,* as mentioned above. Do not offer long supportive conversations; this would impossibly tax your schedule once you had more than one hundred active clients. Instead, ask those callers who call more often to have their questions prepared before they reach you on the phone. Better yet, ask them to leave the prepared question on your voice mail before any background information. This allows you to be available without burning yourself out.

Similarly, forget the strict fifty-minute hour. Prepare your clients for the likelihood that your *session starting time may be flexible,* while explaining that this allows you to extend beyond fifty minutes when necessary. When you give a little more, perhaps your sessions will often be fifty-five minutes. Of course, sessions should not run for an hour and a half, either.

Begin with treatment more than once a month when it is financially possible, but do not worry when it is not. Your clients will still make progress, unless they are in acute crisis. When needs are more urgent, always *begin with more frequency,* explaining to people with financial pressure that they can space out the sessions as soon as the immediate urgency begins to resolve. For clients not in crises, their financial and/or scheduling concerns will usually determine frequency. Certainly, if once a month is useful, biweekly is better, weekly is great, and double sessions are truly the best opportunity for the highest impact. Those who can afford it will benefit from such a more frequent schedule. You will eventually have various clients with each of these types of schedule. *As a highly effective therapist, you can feel ethically comfortable that those who cannot afford more of you will still make good progress.* Your client is doing more of the work, but the needed changes are still happening.

For highest impact, in each session, *start present-focused*. Begin with counseling, drawing the most direct line between where the client is and where he or she wants to be. You can offer this because of a continually growing repertoire of strategies: those you learn about, those you invent, and those that your clients teach you. When clients hit potholes, these show both of you where to dig even deeper and then repair the road.

Glance back to the past to uncover the source of the barriers that have gotten in your client's way. At the end of the session, especially for intermittent clients, summarize what you have both learned and give the client some homework, even if it is only a suggestion to reflect on a part of the session. It helps if you write this down for people—unless your handwriting is like mine, in which case your clients may prefer to write it themselves. And, the very act of their writing it reinforces the new information and perspective.

Even though you may agree with me not to participate in the HMO panels, consider filing outpatient treatment reports (OTRs) for your clients. First, you can describe the advantages and disadvantages of such reports to your clients, especially in terms of privacy. At this point, if someone warns you to avoid some level of specificity, be sure that he or she understands that this may affect the authorization. Leaving this decision to the client, I remain in the helper role, serving my client, rather than becoming part of the insurance establishment.

The Tao Helps Write Your Managed Care OTRs

After years of filing outpatient treatment reports, I have gradually been trained by case reviewers how to write them so the reviewers usually offer more sessions and seldom require my wasting time on "peer review." These days, on the rare occasions that I have to talk to a clinician, I ask the case manager to select one for me who actually has a clinical practice, and preferably not a psychiatrist. Case-review pay is so much less than clinical fees that the psychiatrists who do it are more likely not in practice. Avoiding these clinician interviews and especially with nonpractitioners is a Tao-inspired art—and quite a useful one. My experience with many of the reviewing psychiatrists (as opposed to the case-manager clerks) suggests that the reason they are probably not working in private practice themselves is that they would never be able to build one. This puts you at a disadvantage in two ways. First, these individuals may lack sensitivity to your clients, owing to the same personal qualities of emotional myopia that prevent their attracting their own clients. Second, they may resent you without even knowing you, especially if you are successfully out-of-plan. Therefore, they may seek to devalue your work. When you do have occasion to speak with peer reviewers, you may still apply the strategies outlined below for the greatest effect. However, *your main objective will be to avoid that level of interference by writing reports that allow case reviewers, who are often very nice people, to authorize more sessions.*

Such case reviewers have taught me all the strategies enumerated below. They are often very kind to me. This is mutual. As they are accustomed to irritability from us therapists, the case reviewers feel relieved by warm treatment. A friendly attitude toward these clerks is so refreshing for them that they may have sometimes even felt obligated to explain to me how I missed their criteria. When I did not give them what they needed to approve more sessions, these people would sometimes explain exactly which verbiage would have worked better. How they managed that while speaking over recorded lines impressed me.

Although they would never tell me what to write, *they would simply contrast my presentation with the kinds of wording that would fit their criteria.* Over time, they trained me thoroughly so that I now get compliments from reviewers over my reports. Of course, along the way, my clients paid the price until I learned how to write effective OTRs. Your clients need not pay the same cost, however, as we will now review exactly what I learned.

A handy Aikido element of this approach to OTRs is that you will be working within the insurance industry's medical model. The bad news is that insurance companies do not see any need to reimburse your clients for anything other than mental disorders. However, the force that you can harness is that the insurers "medicalize" normal human experience. Inside the medical model, noble human struggles become rendered pathological. As a result, you can find accurate descriptions for most people's experience that will fit their filter—which is important because case reviewers' computers see only what their filter allows them to see.

The balance we will seek is that of presenting only what is accurate for the case review, while speaking in the terms meaningful to the reviewer's computer program. Once again, our little sails will harness the prevailing winds to serve our clients.

First, understand that managed care case reviewers are trained in utilization review criteria that render "subjective distress" unimportant. Putting it bluntly, they are usually cautioned not to care how our clients feel. Their own supervisors disparage emotional distress as a trivial symptom of the "worried well." So, to fit their criteria, express symptoms in terms of any *impairments of function*. This can include effects on occupation, education, relationships, or self-care. If your client is doing flawlessly well in all these areas, then claim—if it is true—that their functioning will deteriorate if they do not have treatment. Later, we will examine a sample report that details common examples of impairments of function. They are more common than you might think.

Further, consider whether your client has a *complex case.* If so, you may note any personality features that make recovery take longer. We each know relatively few people without some "personality disorder" features. Of course, these features alone would not require treatment, and managed care prefers not to treat personality disorders anyway. However, these features allow an accurate justification for continued treatment, because they hinder recovery from even mild Axis I disorders. This allows gentle diagnoses, often in the 309.xx range, while documenting "medical necessity."

You may be asked about your treatment style. Your case reviewer will not recognize "Aikido treatment." However, he or she is likely to recognize terms such as "a combination of therapeutic stabilization and problem-focused treatment," which you will also find in the sample report. Applying a phenomenal focus, as we have described, qualifies you for this approved orientation.

As for your modality, reviewers are likely to recognize *time-efficient long-term treatment.* This is an approved managed care modality. If the reviewers have not heard of it, refer them to the article by James Sabin, MD, "Time-Efficient Long-Term Psychotherapy in Managed Care," in the *Harvard Review of Psychiatry,* vol. 3, no. 3 (1995), pp. 163–165.

If, despite your efforts, authorization for sessions is cut off, let clients know their options. Of course, they may self-pay. For one session a month, many will decide to do this. Or they can skip a couple of months and then start treatment again. When they do, you can submit an updated OTR, including documentation of any deterioration in function during the break. You must also offer to make a low-cost clinic referral, as well as offering to appeal the HMO decision before the break, if someone is stopping treatment for financial reasons. In addition, to avoid being cut off in the first place, document any natural breaks in treatment—and their effects. The managed care reviewers will usually accept this as demonstrating that the treatment is medically necessary. Finally, after six months of no treatment, most managed care companies consider resumption of sessions a new treatment, allowing for an "initial" report rather than an "update" report.

At the end of this section, you will find a template OTR, which can either function as a model for your own template or assist you in filling out treatment update forms. It is easier to delete or modify parts of an overly inclusive OTR document, which is already on your word processor, than to write a new report each time. For the increasingly prevalent OTR forms, the template provides ready language and options. In the template, you will note my comments set off in brackets.

The following template uses the challenging example of a high-functioning person with only an adjustment disorder diagnosis on Axis I. Interestingly, the report shows how features that people commonly present to us can be applied to indicate medical necessity for treatment. To summarize, we are simply aligning particular forces toward a useful objective:

- ☯ The first force is the challenges common to the human condition, such as those we have noticed in this text.
- ☯ The second force is the shortsightedness of the insurance industry, despite the data showing that outpatient treatment saves them money overall, in trying to make you and your client go away.
- ☯ The objective is to achieve your client's request that you help gain insurance benefits for your work together.

As promised, this happens without fabrications. Again, this is only a template, and probably no one is going to have the entire array of personality symptoms presented in that section. (Further, if someone managed this, but still did not qualify for any single personality disorder, the Axis II classification would be "atypical personality disorder.") Instead, in a normal population, people will often demonstrate one or more features of a single personality disorder. This is enough to "complicate the presentation," and it is just enough to warrant longer treatment.

The particular symptoms in people with just a few dysfunctional personality "features," as opposed to those with a true personality disorder, will often be the less known and milder symptoms. Thus, the listed template examples use such language, including sometimes-overlooked features that would qualify someone for each of the listed complications. Within each paragraph on personality features, I have listed the least pathological criteria that nonetheless justify the presentation of a "personality features" designation, which in turn renders the case complex. If you think back to our courses in psychopathology, these features had us worried ourselves. (As I was writing this, my teenage daughter, with the help of an Internet site that asks questions and tells you everything from what religion you should be to what mental disorder you might have, asked me whether liking some things and disliking others means you have borderline personality disorder.)

The template goes even further in this useful direction as we move into "impairments of function," where we are not limited by the *Diagnostic and Statistical Manual-IV* (DSM-IV) classification system. Our sample includes examples of qualified criteria for impairments of function that are commonly found. A few lesser impairments will elevate the intensity level from mild to moderate. Again, your client is not likely to have all the impairments listed.

The stress criteria mentioned in the template are also helpful examples of factors that show continued need for treatment if they are present. Stress is ubiquitous in contemporary life, and it comes in handy in explaining the necessity for sessions.

As you can see, our dilemma is that we must work within the medical model of human struggles, without which there would be no insurance. However, it would be unfair to categorize people in overly pathological terms. The solution is to ride the momentum of the medical model itself. Because this model sees healthy struggles pathologically, it has terms that can qualify people for help without overdiagnosing them—but you must use these terms. The point is never to fabricate; instead, the point is Aikido. We can present evidence in terms to which managed care reviewers are prepared to listen.

Finally, it is ethically wise to discuss the presentation with your client. There are important privacy issues involved, even though the insurance companies promise not to circulate these reports. As a result, the decision to disclose must always belong fully to our clients. I will often tell a client, "Managed care companies are bound to keep the report private and not even share it with the rest of the insurance company, but we can never be sure. They are allowed to refuse to cover further sessions, under your contract with them, if we don't send this in. On the other hand, they are not allowed to request or use these reports to justify decisions about your future insurance coverage."

What follows is a sample report. The bracketed sections below are explanatory notes and not part of the report:

INITIAL TREATMENT PLAN

[or updated treatment plan]

Date of Report: ____________________________

Patient Name: Hugh Min Condition

Membership #: [always include] ____________________

Health Plan: [also include the name of the employer] ____________

____

Date of Birth: ____________________________

Date of First Visit: ________________________

Diagnosis (DSM-IV)

Axis I: 309.00 Adjustment Disorder with Depressed Mood

Axis II: [We will define these below. If more than one of these apply, the client has an atypical personality disorder.]

006.00 Avoidant Personality Features
011.00 Borderline Personality Features
005.00 Dependent Personality Features
004.00 Histrionic Personality Features
003.00 Narcissistic Personality Features
010.00 Obsessive-Compulsive Personality Features
001.00 Paranoid Personality Features

Axis III: High blood pressure [or any other medical conditions that you know are exacerbated by stress. Many are, if you check the literature.]

Axis IV: Psychosocial stressors: [whatever stressors are applicable. Examples include the following.] Concern over health, marital conflict, threats to employment, poor academic performance, complicated bereavement over death of ____________

Severity: 4 - Severe (enduring circumstances)

Axis V: Current GAF: 45 [check criteria in DSM-IV, but watch for this one. An otherwise effective OTR can be shot down because of an overly high Global Assessment of Functioning scale, despite the preponderance of evidence that the GAF scale is notoriously unreliable between raters.]

Initial Reasons for Treatment The patient, a [age]-year-old [fe]male, entered treatment because of [choose or change:] moderate [or severe] depression, moderate anxiety, severe marital conflict, and severe parent-child conflict, which [s]he has been experiencing following the stress of

____

The interaction of the patient's life-stress and personality features render this a complex presentation.

Description of Symptoms [Choose/change these mood symptoms:] The patient has been experiencing diminished energy, and diminished interest in usual activities. [S]he has further been suffering from excessive, inappropriate guilt, as well as irritable mood and dysphoric mood. Symptoms include impaired concentration, feelings of hopelessness, and diminished interest in being with other people. Finally, [s]he is experiencing psychomotor agitation, and diminished ability to feel pleasure.
[In the next section, if several of the symptoms apply, you must determine, using *DSM-IV*, whether the full disorder is present. It usually will not be.]

The patient shows a generalized pattern of social discomfort associated with exaggeration of risks in doing unfamiliar things, fear of saying something foolish in social situations, concern over showing anxiety in front of others, excessive concern over others' perceptions, being easily hurt when criticized, and hesitancy to become involved with others. [These all are avoidant features.]

The patient shows a generalized pattern of unstable mood, relationships, and identity as evidenced in impulsive and self-defeating behavior, intense and poorly modulated anger expression, persistent feelings of emptiness, and a marked fear of abandonment. [These are borderline features.]

The patient shows a generalized pattern of dependent behavior as manifested in being easily hurt by criticism, often being fearful of rejection or abandonment, going along with others for fear of rejection, offering to do things for others in order to be liked, a lack of self-confidence, and feelings of devastation when a relationship ends. [All dependent features.]

The patient shows a generalized pattern of attention-seeking and emotionally dramatic behavior associated with excessive needs for approval, difficulty tolerating frustration, the need for immediate gratification, and self-centeredness. [The histrionic features.]

The patient shows a generalized pattern of ego inflation, deficient empathy, and hypersensitivity to evaluation associated with overreacting to criticism, the perception that one's own problems are unique, a sense of entitlement, excessive needs for praise and approval, a propensity to take advantage of people, fragile self-esteem, frequent feelings of envy, and a lack of sensitivity to the feelings of others. [Narcissistic features.]

The patient shows a generalized pattern of perfectionistic and rigid behavior associated with difficulty showing warmth and tenderness, excessive need to be in control, an obsession with details and rules, indecisiveness for fear of making a mistake, constricted emotional expression, and difficulty throwing things away. [S]he shows hesitancy in letting others do things, believing they will do it wrong, and has a preoccupation with work to the exclusion of other things. [Obsessive-compulsive features.]

The patient shows a generalized pattern of suspiciousness, as evidenced in an unwillingness to self-disclose, holding grudges, being easily slighted or insulted, hypervigilance, restricted emotionality, seeing hidden meanings in the words and actions of others, expectations that others will exploit or take advantage of him [her], and excessive distrust of the words and actions of others. [Paranoid features.]

Onset and exacerbation of these symptoms appears to be associated with psychosocial stressors: [Reiterate whatever stresses are applicable.]

[Here is the "impairment of function" section, so preferred by managed care systems.]

The patient reports moderate impairment in social functioning as exhibited by increased arguments with family members and/or spouse, social withdrawal, diminished social interaction and activities, and poor judgment in social situations. [Several of these would elevate the presentation to a rating of "severe."]

There is moderate impairment in occupational functioning evidenced by diminished concentration at work, excessive preoccupation with work to the exclusion of other things, confusion or lack of direction regarding career, diminished motivation and initiative, and failure to advance in the job because of symptoms. [Most of these would elevate the presentation to a rating of "severe."]

There is moderate academic dysfunction reflected in failure to complete school assignments, excessive shyness with schoolmates, difficulty remembering school assignments, achievement below intellectual ability, and disinterest and lack of motivation. [Several of these would elevate the presentation to a rating of "severe."]

There is moderate impairment in self-care skills, manifested in inadequate attention to nutritional needs, difficulty having fun, and lack of relaxing/pleasurable activities. [These are among the normal—in the sense of common—symptoms that still qualify for this self-care category.]

Psychological Test Results None.
[Don't worry about that; managed care seldom pays for it, so cannot expect it.]

Mental Status Exam

[This may be a required section, but impairment here is never necessary for authorization.]

The patient's appearance can be characterized as appropriate and well groomed. [S]he is well oriented in all spheres. Memory for recent events is normal. The patient's motor behavior is characterized by psychomotor agitation. Speech is logical and coherent. A negligible degree of conceptual disorganization is evident. Regarding perceptual functioning, hallucinations and delusions are denied and none are evidenced. There is an absence of suspiciousness and [s]he shows no difficulty establishing emotional rapport. Mood is depressed, irritable, and anxious [as applicable]. Affect is appropriate [or blunted or labile]. The tone and content of speech evidences a negligible degree of anger and resentment. Suicidal and homicidal ideation are both absent [unless otherwise].

Prior Treatment Efforts The history does not reveal any psychiatric hospitalizations prior to the present treatment. The patient does not report any prior outpatient treatment efforts [unless otherwise].

Medication

[Case reviewers often want to know why you are not using medication for affective symptoms, if you are not. You can mention that medication is not typically used for the personality features that are making this a complex case. (There is some evidence of medication assisting in borderline personality disorder, especially with psychotic features and self-mutilation.) Adjustment disorders do not require medication, as the stress must be managed, and the patient is expected to return to the premorbid emotional state. For anxiety, all medications are addictive, except antidepressants and buspirone (BuSpar), which is often only mildly helpful. For depression, despite the American Psychiatric Association protocols, the research is split. Half the studies show that psychotherapy alone is as effective as medication, even for severe depression. On the other hand, antidepressants are usually benign and have not been shown to have any irreversible side effects. See the section on "The Aikido of Medication."]

Therapy Modalities Individual therapy: monthly [or weekly, or biweekly] for 50 minutes.

Estimated duration of treatment: for the next six months.
[Managed care companies will seldom authorize more than that, and will not hold you to it as long as the next report justifies treatment. They know that there is no evidence that any therapists can predict the future for any single client.]

Primary Therapeutic Orientation

Cognitive–behavioral treatment
Crisis stabilization as needed
Focused symptom reduction therapy as applicable

Treatment Goals **Short- and Long-Term Goals:**
[Examples related to adjustment disorders follow; for other diagnoses, goals also will follow symptoms.]

Development of alternate coping strategies.
Modification of perspective concerning stressful events.
Reduction of impact of stressors.
A more positive, optimistic outlook.
Restoration of normal energy level.
Increased experience of enjoyment of activities.
Improved ability to think and concentrate.

Treatment Progress

[List any goals from the previous report that have improved.]

The patient shows a negligible degree of resistance to treatment and his [her] motivation is fair. [S]he has difficulty focusing because of affective distress. Response to treatment has been positive but slow owing to the exacerbating effects of the continued environmental stress and the complicating effects of the personality features that retard progress with the Axis I symptoms. The patient is showing gradual progress despite the intermittent scheduling of appointments according to the modality of time-efficient long-term treatment [if so].

The patient requires additional treatment because of the continued presence of stressors, because symptoms persist, because of abiding impairments of function, and because the treatment gains are recent and will deteriorate without further treatment [as applicable].

Name of Provider of Services:

Title: Licensed Psychologist [or other certification]

State/License:

[list certification or license number and the applicable state]

Provider's Signature **Date**

How Your Consent-to-Treat Form Can Help Your Practice

Another important detail of independent practice is the design of your consent-to-treat form. Unlike the HIPAA form, it is not a legal requirement, but risk management advice always includes it. As such, it could easily become defensive and off-putting. You have too much Aikido under your belt by this point, however, to settle for that. This two-sided sheet is your first opportunity to help new clients learn about you. As such, it can include whatever you want to be certain you have told your clients, including how to gauge their expectations of progress. With the right tone, you can expect that people will look forward to working with you after reading it. If nicely designed, it serves a triple function:

- ☯ It informs clients of your policies, as is legally advisable.
- ☯ It provides risk management through the client's written agreement with these policies.
- ☯ It presents the nature of your practice because it illustrates your orientation. As you review the text below, you may notice these three elements interwoven throughout.

SOME INFORMATION ABOUT COUNSELING AND THERAPY

The difference between counseling and therapy. Counseling is most effective when it is a strategic process. It provides guidance toward a goal with the help of broader thinking, new skills, or identification of useful old skills. Meanwhile, therapy glances back to the past to uncover the source of any internal barriers that would prevent the application of the strategies that counseling has identified. Typically, these barriers are very old habits, beliefs, or forms of protection that come into rigid operation during stressful times. Then, ways to move past these barriers can be designed. In this way, counseling and therapy are complementary.

Confidentiality. See HIPAA summary for currently mandated federal regulations.

Other ethical expectations. I will accept my client's challenges with unconditional positive regard, or else I must refer that person elsewhere. I may offer to treat various members of a family or other partnership. If so, I will seek to understand conflicting perspectives without bias or taking sides. This maximizes the information available for resolution. On the other hand, if any party feels it is no longer acceptable, I will suggest appropriate referral. I cannot give advice on which goals to hold, but can give concrete direction on how to attain goals and make changes. I am also not permitted to enter into any secondary relationship with a client. Although this rule prevents business dealings and outside friendships, its main purpose is to protect clients from potential exploitation.

—1—

Why I do not participate in HMO panels. To join or not to join, that was my question. Most practitioners dislike HMOs, seeing them as profit-oriented, not care-oriented. Psychologists typically join out of fear of not maintaining a practice, but seldom for any other reason. In contrast, I decided that I was in the business of helping people make brave transformations, and I could not do that as well if I succumbed to such fears in my own life. People who see me decide that what I offer is worth the choice of an out-of-plan person, as our sessions are "cost effective" in terms of the amount we accomplish and the usefulness of the work we do. In addition, I can fight for more sessions from the insurance company without fear of having my contract canceled. So—bottom line—I commit to providing a better value for my clients, which is how I can stay out.

Who benefits from counseling and therapy? Those who benefit from sessions come to work on themselves. Although these people may spend some time noticing the external barriers in their lives, they spend more of their time looking for new internal solutions. In addition, they are open and completely honest in stating their situation and concerns. They identify and focus on their most pressing challenges for the therapist. Finally, they have overcome their ambivalence about changing their lives, and are eager to grow past their difficulties.

People who do not yet take these attitudes still may progress. The process just becomes longer as the therapist and life's distress both guide them toward taking these more practical approaches.

—2—

GENERAL INFORMATION

The nature of this practice. Although this is a general practice, I have a particular interest, which concerns the effects of stress and crisis. Stressful events set in motion old, confining habits of thought, emotion, and behavior. This is a typical occurrence, even in completely normal individuals. If a way can be found to interrupt these old, rigid patterns, then most people can expect to function the way they would prefer. Whether I treat anxiety, depression, family communication problems, or self-esteem issues, it will usually include this perspective.

Appointment times. Appointments are 50 minutes in length. They begin 10 minutes after the scheduled time. This practice allows me to extend more easily beyond 50 minutes when necessary.

The answering system. You can call the office anytime, 24 hours a day, 365 days a year. While I am in the office, I will usually check in hourly. Outside my office hours, I will check in within the next 24 hours. I encourage people to call me with questions, and I am happy to call back. Please be aware that I do not provide emergency services, so circumstances may delay my return call. I will arrange to have emergency services made available on request.

Changing appointments. You can cancel or reschedule your appointment time. In fact, our first meeting probably occurred during an appointment time that someone else had canceled. However, I ask that people give me a few days' notice of cancellations. This way, I have time to contact people, and they have time to adjust their schedules. If I receive less than one full business day's notice, that is, before 9:00 a.m. on the business day preceding the appointment, I must charge you for the time if I do not fill it.

—3—

Insurance and fees. I do not currently raise my fee to reflect demand for my services, but only to reflect changes in the consumer price index. "Point of service" group insurance policies will pay a portion of the services of a licensed psychologist, after you meet your deductible. If they have a list of contracted providers, they may limit the "usual and customary fee" to the amount that these psychologists agreed to accept. HMOs typically will pay nothing. You can pay only the uncovered part of the fee at the session. After you fill out your form, my billing service will file it for you and submit the bill. If there is any balance after insurance and your payments, it is due in full when the bill is received. After thirty (30) days, any bills not paid in full are subject to eighteen (18) percentage points of interest (1.5% per month). In the event that a bill is unpaid, I will add attorneys' fees, collection costs, and interest.

Snow, illness, or emergency cancellations. I understand that you may need to stay home if you believe that traveling would endanger you. I would never wish for you to take a health risk in order to come to the office. With the rare exception of a state-declared snow emergency, I will be here if you decide to come in a storm. If you stay home for snow, illness, or emergencies, we will have a session using Skype or the telephone. On an exceptional basis, I find that this works very well. Or you can cancel as described above under "changing appointments."

I have read both sides of this form and find it acceptable.

______________________________ __________

(Signed) **Date**

— 4 —

As you can see, this form informs clients about the nature of my practice format. I originated it out of concern for items I might forget to tell people new to my practice. Later, when I learned that I should have a consent-to-treat form, I realized that I already had one, and I just needed to add a signature line to it. It also protects me by clarifying my policies according to my understanding of the recommendations of risk management advisors. Still, these are not the greatest benefit of this form. The form also balances the pendulemia of promotional marketing on one hand and dry legalisms on the other. In rhythmic balance, it shows both features and benefits of my services. The response of most potential clients is to want to use the services that the form describes.

One of the items mentioned on the form is a particularly important area to keep to keep in mind in establishing this style of practice, which is that the therapist must deal with bias. The question of bias is primary to whether or not you decide to treat entire families. We turn to this question next.

Why Working with Clients' Family and Friends Works Best

It is natural to feel irritated at some of the treatment your client gets at the hands of other people in his or her life. However, in the same manner as humorist Will Rogers described strangers as friends he had not yet met, your client's family and friends are clients you have not yet treated. It is so routine for many therapists to refuse to work with clients' relatives and friends that many people think this is an ethical rule, and you may have even learned this in your training. You will also note from the aforementioned consent material that this is untrue.

Ethical standards, at least for psychologists, explicitly state that you can choose to treat related individuals, as long as you tell people initially how you work and give the initial client an option to forbid your treatment of relatives and close friends. There are two advantages to working with the client's family and friends. First, it allows you to see a more complete picture and to help much more directly. Additionally, it removes what would otherwise comprise an unnecessary barrier to client referral, which is helpful for this style of practice, as it relies on word-of-mouth rather than selection from a "participating providers" list.

The essential challenge is to deal with any source of bias. Perhaps you can already understand the struggle of clients you have not yet met. Can you put one foot in their lives, too? *If we cannot, ought we to be working with our original clients on this area?* In other words, if I operate from a biased position, I am not useful in the realm of bias, whether or not I treat the friend or relative directly. On the other hand, if I am able to see the validity even in conflicting concerns, then everyone will gain by my working with both parties.

Do Not Discount Your Fees

The Tao of your psychotherapy practice gives you the option to develop a truly independent practice, as we have seen. After noting the advantages of this to your clients, I have suggested that you could elect to build it gradually, if you wish. Doing so would bring an additional detail for you to decide, which is how to set your session fees.

My advice about fees is simple: *Do not discount them.* Why? First, if you want to discount, then your clients would be better off if you work through their HMOs. That way, they would get a better financial arrangement. Second, if you are not worth whatever your fee is, then you should change it. Otherwise, it is better to present a model to others of being paid what one is worth.

I am not suggesting overcharging, of course. As you read in my consent-to-treat form, I raise my fee only in response to increases in the consumer price index, which has left it an average fee all these years. I am just cautioning you against the opposite mistake, which would be to try to lower your fee to fill your caseload.

In response to their recognition that you provide excellent help, your clients will use you as they would any resource, investing in your services to the extent that they value your contribution toward achieving their life goals. In a free-market economy, it is simple to find out one's worth in the marketplace—it is the price that people are willing to pay when they have other choices.

There are other reasons to avoid fee discounts. One of these is best explained with a story. The anecdote is about the famous and talented cartoonist Jules Feiffer, and comes to me via my friend Arthur Kurzweil.

It seems that Feiffer, a then-unknown cartoonist, sent an unsolicited cartoon to the *Village Voice,* thinking that his work might fit the paper's style. Sure enough, he received a call from an editor at the paper, along with an offer. The conversation went something like this:

> "Mr. Feiffer, we liked the cartoons, and would like to use some. We also believe that the *Voice* would be a nice showcase for you as an unknown. We'd be willing to pay you an honorarium of ten dollars per cartoon."
>
> "Thank you for the offer," replied Feiffer, "but actually I think I will donate the cartoons for now."
>
> "Oh, are you financially independent?"
>
> "Not at all. I could use the money."
>
> "Then why not take it?"
>
> "Well, if I donate my cartoons to you, then I am a philanthropist. If I accept your fee, then I am a ten-dollar cartoonist."

Thus, do some pro bono work if you can. You will get more joy from such a gift of yourself than you get from getting paid. But, when it comes to getting paid, please do not discount yourself.

Overcoming Pendulemia Regarding Advertising

To help people find you, it is useful to list yourself in the "yellow pages" in both print and electronic media. You can also list your practice interests, so you get the right calls. The balance here is to provide enough information so prospective clients can see the scope of your interests, without placing an overly large display ad. In my own local print listing I always mentioned the following three practice interests (I am using the past tense, because, after many years, I started to just list my web site, nothing else):

- Treating stress, anxiety, and depression.
- Communication for couples and families.
- Self-esteem enhancement.

If it is too large, the ad will convey the wrong message, which is either that you are a group practice or that you need to spend more than others do in order to attract clients. Listing your practice by your personal name rather than by a business name also clearly shows you as an individual practitioner. Many private-pay clients tend to want the privacy of a solo practice. A crowded waiting room might look impressive for a physician, but can be inconvenient for many psychotherapy clients, a few of whom might be embarrassed and more of whom will want to use waiting time to prepare their thoughts without the distraction of a busy waiting room. So, in the same way that you probably prefer a separate exit from your office entrance, you will be better off listing yourself in a small display ad and using your name. Finally, consider using your nickname if you consider it appropriate, which gives prospective clients a clue that you have a peer attitude. At least in the United States, a psychotherapy consumer is likely to feel more invited to call Bill than William. Of course, if everyone calls you "William," then that is your familiar name as well.

When you receive each directory call, you have an opportunity to present your practice style immediately. If this person becomes your client, you are building the relationship from this moment. You can begin in this initial conversation to develop rapport and offer support. Next is a step-by-step script that fulfills both opportunities when responding to a caller.

> First, congratulate the caller for the choice to make these calls.
>
> "Well, you've made the right start. Calling around as you are doing now will give you a sense of how people speak with you before you make an appointment to meet with anyone." [The next part offers a set of suggestions and comprises a work sample.]
>
> "Would it be okay if I give you some advice on how to search for a therapist? [The answer to this question is always "yes."] This will also give you a sense on what I think is important. First, see how they treat you on the phone, whether they talk down to you or not, whether you feel comfortable. Don't blame yourself if you don't feel comfortable. You can expect people to act pretty much the same in their offices.
>
> "Second, ask them some question about strategy. It's one thing to understand, and another to know how to help. You could phrase this by asking if they take a practical approach or if they help direct you to your goals, or if they are strategic.
>
> "Now, when you are listening to their answers, there are a couple of extremes to avoid. Some people—though this is rare—sound like they want to run your life. Others might say something to the effect that they will facilitate you or ask the right questions, which is a passive approach. What is better, from my point of view, is someone who says they can guide you, but that you'll be in charge of the direction. That's

as much as you can find out on the phone. Then, it takes a visit to see if they can deliver on what they promised."

This will often intrigue the caller enough to want to see you. More and more, you will not have to advertise your practice, as clients will be drawn to you. Your reputation for fine work will act as a magnet to your practice.

Once more, you can see that we are creating a rhythmic Aikido balance between the extremes of unprofessionally overt marketing and self-effacing shyness about the efficacy of our coaching. This also models a similar balance for the self-esteem of our clients.

Because information about them is mailed and e-mailed to us, one can easily find workshops on how to promote professional referrals, how to write letters of introduction, and how to advertise most effectively. There are also home-study programs. I do not doubt that marketing approaches can produce results. They just do not interest me; client-to-client referrals are more reliable over time. They are also a lot more enjoyable than "farming" relationships with marginally interested doctors whom you have cold-called. When clients refer their friends to you, you just have to avoid ruining the rapport they already bring as soon as they walk in. This is where we would prefer to live and work. In special cases, however, doctor referrals can be equally enjoyable—if they come from sharp and caring physicians who have picked up on your usefulness with one of their patients. These top doctors usually have such a good rapport with patients that their referrals are almost as warm as ones that come from friends.

Additional Ways to Diversify and Express Yourself

I often tell my clients that I am in the "more" school of change. I expect that they will agree with me that it is better to add than to subtract. The Tao of your psychotherapy practice fits this preference. It is not necessary to sacrifice much to develop a managed-care-resistant style of practice. Mostly, *you need only to abandon the set of reasons with which you have been telling yourself that it is impossible.* I became immune to managed care by accident—yet you can similarly inoculate yourself deliberately. The cost of this vaccination is minimal. Your model, your more frequent clients, your HMO participation—none of these must be discarded immediately, if ever. Seen in this way, the intermittent, the TELT treatment that we mentioned above is just a way of adding diversification to your practice. In this section, we will briefly review additional ways of diversifying your practice, as these could also promote additional freedom in your career. In addition, any independent sources of revenue would provide more freedom in your practice choices. Many therapists have developed additional specializations. This so-called niche marketing allows one to meet an unfilled need for treatment.

A couple of additional caveats to note: First, do not pick any area that you do not love. Presumably, we did not enter this field just for its income benefits. There are several easier ways to make much higher incomes than we ever can. At best, we are essentially well-paid hourly workers. Thus, it is important that we not ruin our love of being a psychotherapist en route to finding a greater market for our services.

Second, adopting a specialty sets up a separate, higher standard of care for your practice. This is a risk-management issue. Certainly find additional training in the niche area, but avoid calling yourself a specialist unless a clear standard of care is available and has been mastered. You may have noticed that the first words I use to describe my practice on the consent form are "This is a general practice." This is specifically to avoid this legal issue. This caveat can also be managed by using different language, such as "interest in" or "practice in."

Having said all that, some additional specializations include the following:

1. *Special population interests,* such as rehabilitation issues, chronic disease, chronic pain, disabilities, geriatrics, ethnic populations, infertility, sexual dysfunction, divorce, trauma recovery, substance abuse, blended families, bereavement, impulse control disorders, athletes, eating disorders, and violent abusers.

2. *Special practice interests,* such as stress management, "wellness" programs, parenting training, forensics, corporate team building, executive coaching (personal counseling for those in business settings), career planning, group therapy, motivational speaking, and hypnosis.

3. Some therapists have moved into *crossover fields*. For these therapists, the additional revenue provides some financial independence, which in turn provides some more freedom in the course of developing independent practice. Participation in crossover fields is different from doing psychotherapy with a special population, because it entails activities other than psychotherapy. Popular crossover fields include divorce mediation and bodywork, both of which require additional training, but can be successful.

MDs and nurse-practitioner psychotherapists also have the option of prescribing medication. In addition, they often find work providing psychotropic medication backup for nonmedical psychotherapists. Further, some psychologists' organizations are exploring winning this prescription privilege for psychologists.

I have some doubt whether this is a useful direction for psychologists. In questioning this direction, I am questioning not the usefulness of medication, as we have discussed, but of combining psychotherapy and medication management in the same practice. In other words, I am an advocate for what is called *split treatment*. The early tradition of combined treatment has actually hurt the image of psychiatrists. This is part of the reason that they have a somewhat less favorable public perception than do nonmedical psychotherapists. To the population that prefers psychological change to medication, they are seen as pill-pushers, whereas we psychologists are seen as helpful. Second, HMOs have largely relegated psychiatric practice to medication, even when psychiatrists have other training. Because the HMOs would rather remunerate medication than psychotherapy in most cases, a move to have nonphysicians prescribe would be an opportunity for further HMO restrictions on psychotherapy. This would be a sad outcome for the affected therapists, and especially for their clients.

Another form of business diversification is the opportunity to offer seminars either for other therapists or for the general public. These are quite different from each other, of course. If you have an area of expertise that you would enjoy offering in a seminar format, you can either work for an educational company or market it yourself. You know, by the frequency at which you receive mailings about various seminars, that continuing education comprises a growing industry. You can find a range of companies in this field quite easily, by noticing the organizations that currently market to you.

Presenting seminars for the public is a very useful form of self-marketing. One can secure free rooms at colleges, churches, libraries, and schools, as well as free advertising in newspapers, because these are public service activities. Pick something you already know a great deal about, which your existing clients love to hear about.

For additional ideas, look at the special populations and special practice interests listed previously. Enjoy yourself, making it a win–win situation. You will enjoy offering to new people the insights you have learned, and at the same time you are expanding awareness of your work.

Finally, one of the most effective ways of contributing your insights to colleagues and the public is through the medium that you are reading right now. Because of exciting developments in technology, the publishing world has been moving past the pendulemia of previous decades.

In the past, an author had two dichotomous choices: find a publisher or print through a "vanity press." Arthur Kurzweil, who has extensive publishing experience, including being vice president and editor-in-chief of Jason Aronson, Inc. when it offered the Behavioral Science Book Club, expressed the change to me by stating, "The playing field has been leveled as never before." Writing under contract with a publishing house can be a good arrangement for a well-known author, but not so for a new one. Publishers pin their financial hope on finding those few bestsellers that take off, but they do not know how to locate or create them. As Kurzweil states, "If they knew how, they would do it more often." Instead, publishers supply high-quality developmental editing, copyediting, and proofreading when they place a bet on a new author. In return for this, they assume ownership of the work, supplying the author with commissions of about 5 percent for book sales. Marketing, if it is to occur, is left up to the author in most cases.

Two developments have changed the options for authors: printing-on-demand technology, which allows affordable printing as orders are placed, and the Internet as a setting for publicizing projects. As a result, if you believe you have a book in you, once you have written it, you can easily enter the independent world of self-publishing. The balanced options available can be in the best tradition of Tao harmony. For instance, with Paradoxical Press, you would affordably contract for the same quality of editing and printing expertise as a publishing house would provide, while retaining full ownership of your work. In addition, its marketing department offers what a traditional house would not: a marketing plan tailored to your own preferences. Finally, because you retain ownership of your work, even modest book sales should recap your investment.

Writing, along with seminars and diversification, can become wonderful vehicles for making people aware of you and growing your psychotherapy practice, as long as they follow the essential Tao principle: *You are riding the motivating wave of your own interests.* In other words, when you are aflame with the love of your own opportunities for contribution, people become interested in watching the illumination you give off.

5

Where Would You Like to Go?

Where Would You Like to Go?

We have learned together how Tao-inspired insights, especially in their Aikido version, allow us to harness the forces hindering our practices to our advantages. Surprisingly:

- The power of managed care can place us in the correct stress-level range to provide our best services.
- Our personal struggles and successes with our own versions of the human condition become the context for a powerful therapeutic alliance.
- The natural forces resisting change in our clients can be harnessed through specific therapeutic strategies in the tune of Aikido and through an earnest, peer attitude.
- Extreme polarities can be harmonized without losing the energies offered by either side. This applies equally to client dilemmas, practice orientation, and marketing decisions.
- Even the confusing lack of normalization in the field of psychology becomes an ally, as we take a phenomenal focus that applies the best of each of the theories to the phases of brain function they best serve. In this manner, the phenomenon of

> the state-rigidity stress–regress becomes a theoretical hub on which to achieve psychotherapy integration.

So, now you have your boat, your sail, and effective techniques for sailing. Where would you like to go?

In my career as a psychologist, I have met some financially successful, self-made individuals who began with no financial advantages at all. Sometimes they also came from very unsupportive homes. Yet they built impressive financial achievements.

I appreciated that success in this handful of people, but I paid little attention to it, because people come to me to discuss what does not work in their lives. No one makes an appointment with me to work on his or her amazing financial success. As I focused on their areas of difficulty, I noticed only peripherally that they all had something fascinating in common.

The first time I worked with one of these people, I wondered how the session would go. After all, I was meeting him during a time of stress for him, and he was accustomed to being a master of his universe—I knew this because of his very public accomplishments. However, I need not have worried. He was completely open to my contributions, and once he saw that I had skill in my field, he openly craved my input. This was a relief, but I have good relationships with almost all of my clients, so I thought about it no further.

The second person had quite extraordinary wealth. Thus, once again, I wondered whether this person would use this as a barrier to benefiting from a non-wealthy therapist. Again, it was no issue. His nickname for me was "Coach." The third such person had built a very successful company single-handedly. When I noted with delight that he had the same receptivity, I finally saw the pattern.

These were all men, you will note. Men are not the most likely to admit confusion and allow someone else to be the expert. However, these men were the least defensive of any male clients I had ever met. A friend of one of them once mentioned that she knew from him that he was my client and volunteered how he had learned to become so successful. Without prompting from me, she confirmed what I now suspected. He had shown the same wide-open receptivity, the same "coachability," in finding mentors who could show him how to make money.

Thus, in addition to the well-known quality of *follow-through*, we can add this second quality of *receptivity* to coaching as an essential factor of success. There are exceptions, of course. My understanding is that some men find remarkable success by being remarkably unscrupulous, remarkably workaholic, or both. However, I do not meet these men in my office too often. My clients attempt to keep their souls intact, and, for them, success requires being very open to coaching.

In this and many other ways, life has taught me that "you don't know what you don't know." I feel fascinated whenever I learn something important, valuable, and new. *Half the fascination is how thoroughly unaware I was that the new learning even existed to be learned.*

You are now in a position to benefit from the measure of this trait in yourself. You have read about a wide-ranging and innovative practice approach. In doing so, you have read about specific techniques with the rationale that they will heighten your effectiveness—and this has been the mildest part of the presentation. To serve the cause of professional independence, you have read about phenomena that challenge the tendency of our past professional training to separate us from our clients. Further, you have read about an ancient philosophical metaphor, which we invoked with the claim that it can help transform your clients' lives—and yours along the way. No matter whether you tend to be left-brained or right-brained, at least some of this is likely to seem foreign. Yet here you are.

Therefore, you probably have the data to know how coachable you are choosing to be. The days to come will also allow you to benefit from your skill in follow-through. Recall the story of our first metaphorical Aikido therapist, the biblical father Jacob. As therapists, we seldom give direct advice on where someone should go, so it means something to us when we do so. I am advising you: Do not let go of whatever attacks you without wresting a blessing from it. Although you may have thought differently—although most of your colleagues will insist differently—this is the best of all times to be a psychotherapist. *People are seeking purpose, reliable change, and freedom in their lives, and they are increasingly aware that we might be helpful in that regard.*

Decide to make your practice work; make it full and fulfilling. Construct it free of constraints, and insist that every obstacle become an opportunity. Your clients need this from you; your quality of work and your quality of life require it as well.

Bibliography

Note: The following bibliography, in addition to referencing citations from the previous text, includes references documenting the phenomena we have been discussing in more depth. Most of this research is quite old. For example, inverted-U research tapered off after the phenomenon become obvious and accepted. The state-rigidity research is likewise rather dated because it was inspired by interest in rigid thinking as it relates to authoritarianism, which was occasioned by the horrors of World War II. In addition, this state-rigidity research eventually tapered off, perhaps for the same reason as the inverted-U research, or perhaps because psychological theories failed to adequately model it.

Andreasen, N. J., Noyes, R. Jr., and Hartford, C. E. Factors influencing adjustment of burn patients during hospitalization. In A. Monat and R. Lazarus (eds.), *Stress and Coping.* New York: Columbia University Press, 1977.

Arkes, H. R., and Garske, J. P. *Psychological Theories of Motivation.* Monterey, CA: Brooks/Cole Publishers, 1977.

Bandler, R., and Grinder, J. *Structure of Magic: I.* Palo Alto, CA: Science and Behavior Books, 1975.

Barthol, R. P., and Ku, N. D. Regression under stress to first learned behavior. In G. Lindzey, C. Hall, and M. Manosevitz (eds.), *Theories of Personality: Primary Sources and Research*. New York: John Wiley & Sons, 1973.

Beam, J. C. Serial learning and conditioning under real life stress. *Journal of Abnormal and Social Psychology,* 1955;51:543–552.

Beier, E. G. The effect of induced anxiety on flexibility of intellectual functioning. *Psychological Monographs,* 1951;65(9) (Whole No. 326).

Berne, E. *Transactional Analysis in Psychotherapy.* New York: Grove, 1961.

Bernstein, S. A time-saving technique for the treatment of simple phobias. *American Journal of Psychotherapy,* 1999;53:501–512.

Bettelheim, B. Individual and mass behavior in extreme situations. *Journal of Abnormal and Social Psychology,* 1943;38:417–452.

Broadbent, D. E. *Decision and Stress.* New York: Academic Press, 1971.

Castonguay, L. G., et al. Integrative cognitive therapy for depression: A preliminary investigation. *Journal of Psychotherapy Integration,* 2004;14:4–20.

Chaplin, J. P., and Krawiec, T. S. *Systems and Theories of Psychology.* New York: Holt, Rinehart, & Winston, 1960.

Child, I. L. *Humanistic Psychology and the Research Tradition: Their Several Virtues.* New York: John Wiley & Sons, 1973.

Chown, S. M. Rigidity—A flexible concept. *Psychological Bulletin,* 1959;56:195–223.

Cowen, E. L. The influence of varying degrees of psychological stress on problem-solving rigidity. *Journal of Abnormal and Social Psychology,* 1952;47:512–519.

Csikszentmihalyi, M. *Flow: The Psychology of Optimal Experience.* New York: Harper & Row, 1990.

Dittes, J. E. Impulsive closure and failure-induced threat. *Journal of Abnormal and Social Psychology,* 1961;63:562–569.

Duffy, E., *Activation and Behavior.* New York: John Wiley & Sons, 1962.

Easterbrook, J. A. The effect of emotion on cue utilization and the organization of behavior. *Psychological Review,* 1959;66:183–201.

Folkman, S., Schaefer, C., and Lazarus, R. S. Cognitive processes as mediators of stress and coping. In V. Hamilton and D. M. Warburton, *Human Stress and Cognition: An Information Processing Approach.* New York: John Wiley & Sons, 1979.

Frankl, V. *Man's Search for Meaning.* Boston: Beacon Press, 2000.

Gardner, H. *Extraordinary Minds: Portraits of 4 Exceptional Individuals and an Examination of our Own Extraordinariness.* New York: Basic Books, 1997.

Grinker, R. R., and Spiegel, J. P. *Men under Stress.* Philadelphia: Blakiston, 1945.

Hull, C. L. *Principles of Behavior.* New York: Appleton-Century-Crofts, 1943.

Isen, A. M., Shalker, T. E., Clark, M., and Karp, L. Affect, accessibility of material in memory, and behavior: a cognitive loop? *Journal of Personality and Social Psychology,* 1978;36: 1–11.

Kemeny, J. G. *The Need for Change: The Legacy of TMI.* Washington, DC: The President's Commission on the Accident at Three Mile Island, 1979.

Kendig, I. Studies in perseveration: IV. Selective perseveration and repetition. *Journal of Psychology,* 1936;3:253–259.

Kobasa, S. C. Stressful life events, personality, and health: An inquiry into hardiness. *Journal of Personality and Social Psychology,* 1979;37:1–11.

Kuhn, T.S. *The Essential Tension: Selected Studies in Scientific Tradition and Change.* Chicago: University of Chicago Press, 1977.

Kuhn, T.S. *The Structure of Scientific Revolutions.* Chicago: University of Chicago Press, 1996.

Lacey, J. Somatic response patterning and stress. In M. H. Appley and R. Trumball (eds.), *Psychological Stress.* New York: Appleton–Century–Crofts, 1967.

Lambert, M. J., and Barley, D. E. Research summary on the therapeutic relationship and psychotherapy outcome. *Psychotherapy,* 2001;38:357–361.

LeDoux, Joseph. *The Emotional Brain: The Mysterious Underpinnings of Emotional Life.* New York: Touchstone Books, 1998.

Lloyd, P. E., and Dicken, P. *Location in Space: A Theoretical Approach to Economic Geography.* New York: Harper and Row, 1972.

Maddi, S. R. *Personality Theories: A Comparative Analysis* (rev. ed.). Homewood, IL: Dorsey, 1972.

Malone, T. B., Kirkpatrick, M., and Mallory, K. Human factors evaluation of control room design and operator performance at Three Mile Island. Alexandria, VA: The Essex Corporation, 1980 (NTIS No. NUREG/CR-1270).

Markman, H., Stanley, S., and Blumberg, S. *Fighting for Your Marriage: Positive Steps for Preventing Divorce and Preserving a Lasting Love.* New York: Jossey-Bass, 1994.

McCormick, E. J. *Human Factors in Engineering and Design.* New York: McGraw-Hill, 1976.

Mechanic, D. Some modes of adaptation: defense. In A. Monat and R. Lazarus (eds.), *Stress and Coping.* New York: Columbia University Press, 1977.

Meichenbaum, D. *Cognitive-Behavior Modification.* New York: Plenum, 1977.

Pally, S. Cognitive rigidity as a function of threat. *Journal of Personality,* 1955;23:346–355.

Patrick, J. R. Studies in rational behavior and emotional excitement: II. The effect of emotional excitement on rational behavior in human subjects. *Journal of Comparative Psychology,* 1934;18:153–195.

Phillips, L., and Smith, J. G. *Rorschach Interpretation: Advanced Technique.* New York: Grune and Stratton, 1953.

Phillips, M. *The Seven Laws of Money.* New York: Random House, 1974.

Postman, L., and Bruner, J. S. Perception under stress. *Psychological Review,*1948;55:314–323.

Rogers, C. R. *On Becoming a Person: A Therapist's View of Psychotherapy.* Boston: Houghton Mifflin, 1961.

Rokeach, M. Generalized mental rigidity as a factor in ethnocentrism. *Journal of Abnormal and Social Psychology,* 1948;40:259–278.

Rokeach, M. The effect of perception time upon rigidity and concreteness of thinking. *Journal of Experimental Psychology,* 1950;40:206–216.

Ronan, W. W. *Training for Emergency Procedures in Multiengine Aircraft.* Pittsburgh: American Institute for Research, 1953.

Royce, J. R. Metaphoric knowledge and humanistic psychology. In J. F. T. Bugental (ed.), *Challenges of Humanistic Psychology.* New York: McGraw-Hill, 1967, p. 21.

Sabin, J. E. Time-efficient long-term psychotherapy in managed care. *Harvard Review of Psychiatry,* 1995;3:163–165.

Sargent, T. O., and Blum, R. B. Predicting and controlling performance shaping factors. *Transactions of the American Nuclear Society.* La Grange Park, IL: American Nuclear Society, 1980 (NTIS No. TANSAO 34 1-899 1080).

Shiffrin, R. M., and Schneider, W. Controlled and automatic human information processing: II. Perceptual learning, automatic attending, and a general theory. *Psychological Review,* 1977;84:127–190.

Smock, C. D. The influence of psychological stress on the intolerance of ambiguity. *Journal of Abnormal and Social Psychology,* 1955(a);50:177–182.

Smock, C. D. The influence of stress on the perception of incongruity. *Journal of Abnormal and Social Psychology,* 1955(b);50:354–356.

Spaulding, R. C., and Ford, C. V. The Pueblo incident: Psychological reactions to the stresses of imprisonment and repatriation. *American Journal of Psychiatry,* 1972;129:17–26.

Spence, K. W. *Behavior Theory and Conditioning.* New Haven, CT: Yale University Press, 1956.

Suzuki, D. T. *Zen and Japanese Culture.* New York: MJF Books, 1997.

Ullman, L. P., and Krasner, L. *A Psychological Approach to Abnormal Behavior.* Englewood Cliffs, NJ: Prentice-Hall, 1969.

Wandersman, A., Poppen, P., and Ricks, D. *Humanism and Behaviorism: Dialogue and Growth.* New York: Pergamon, 1976.

Wolpe, J. *Psychotherapy by Reciprocal Inhibition*. Stanford, CA: Stanford University Press, 1958.

Yankelovich, D. *New Rules*. New York: Random House, 1981.

Zajonc, R. B. Social facilitation. *Science,* 1965;149:269–274.

Zajonc, R. B. Feeling and thinking: Preferences need no inferences. *American Psychologist,* 1980;35(2):151–175.

Index

About the Author

Dr. Rick Blum, a licensed psychologist in West Hartford, Connecticut, has enjoyed a full-time psychotherapy practice since 1986. With degrees from Brandeis University, the University of Iowa, and Syracuse University, he received his PhD. from Saybrook University. Saybrook University, whose founders included luminaries Abraham Maslow and Carl Rogers, and with faculty such as Rollo May and Sam Keen, is the leading graduate institute in what is known as the "third force" of psychology, devoted to the achievement of personal freedom and offers a humanistic approach as an alternative to psychoanalytic and behaviorist perspectives. For a decade Dr. Blum was the director of the Change Agents Training Institute, providing joint Masters degrees with Fairfield University, and later with Vermont College of Norwich University. Dr. Blum has also distinguished himself in his private practice by earning a reputation for remarkable results, allowing him to be one of the few psychologists with a brimming schedule without entering any managed care panels. For many years, in addition to his private practice, Dr. Blum has been a consultant and teacher for a wide range of municipal and corporate clients.

Made in the USA
Monee, IL
13 September 2026

62980996R00132